Recapturing Competence

A System's Change for Geropsychiatric Care

The contributions of **Gail S. Fidler, OTR, FAOTA**, to the fields of Mental Health and Occupational Therapy have earned her recognition throughout the United States and abroad. Her consultation, workshops, and lectures have spanned a breadth of issues including health systems management, supervision, the teaching–learning process, human performance and purposeful activity, group process, leadership, and professional development.

Gail Fidler serves as visiting Professor, College Misericordia, the latest in a list of appointments that have included New York University, Columbia University, San Jose State University, Boston University, University of Pennsylvania and Kean College. Her long and abiding commitment to quality treatment for the mentally ill is reflected in the service positions she has held, which include chief executive officer, Hagadorn Center for Geriatrics; rehabilitation consultant at the New Jersey Division of Mental Health and Hospitals as well as at the Maryland Department of Health and Mental Hygiene; management and clinical positions in occupational therapy for the Veterans Administration in Army, state, and proprietary hospitals. Gail Fidler has previously authored the widely used text *Design of Rehabilitation Services in Psychiatric Hospital Settings*, two landmark occupational therapy texts, and numerous professional papers. She has received many awards and honors for her contributions to the field of occupational therapy and mental health. Her undergraduate degree was received from Lebanon Valley College and her graduate work in occupational therapy was completed at the University of Pennsylvania.

Barbara J. Bristow, MSW, has devoted more than a decade of her career to the field of Gerontology. As an assistant hospital administrator and executive assistant for the Hagadorn Center for Geriatrics, she played an active role in the conversion of the facility to a geropsychiatric treatment and rehabilitation hospital. During her tenure with the New Jersey Division of Mental Health and Hospitals and the Department of Human Services, Barbara Bristow was instrumental in implementing a continuum of services for the elderly state-hospital patients, focusing on their placement in private nursing homes, implementing and monitoring a case-management system aimed at reducing unnecessary hospital or other institutional care of the elderly. Barbara Bristow received her Baccalaureate degree from the University of California, Santa Barbara, and her Master's Degree in Social Work from Rutgers University, New Jersey.

RECAPTURING COMPETENCE

A System's Change for Geropsychiatric Care

Gail S. Fidler

in collaboration with

Barbara J. Bristow

SPRINGER PUBLISHING COMPANY
New York

Springer Publishing Company, Inc.
536 Broadway
New York, NY 10012-3955

92 93 94 95 96/5 4 3 2 1

Library of Congress Cataloging-in-Publication Data

Fidler, Gail S.
Recapturing competence : a system's change for geropsychiatric care / Gail S. Fidler, in collaboration with Barbara Bristow.
p. cm.
Includes bibliographical references and index.
ISBN 0-8261-7760-3
1. Aged—Mental health services—New Jersey—Case studies.
2. Mentally ill aged—Institutional care—New Jersey—Case studies.
3. Psychiatric hospitals—New Jersey—History—20th century.
4. Geriatric psychiatry. I. Bristow, Barbara. II. Title.
[DNLM: 1. Hospitals, Psychiatric—organization & administration.
2. Mental Disorders—in old age. 3. Mental Disorders—rehabilitation. 4. Mental Health Services—organization & administration. WM 30 F451r]
RC451.4A5F54 1992
618.97'689—dc20
DNLM/DLC
for Library of Congress 91-4998
CIP

Printed in the United States of America

The opinions and concepts expressed in this work are those of the author's and do not necessarily represent those of the New Jersey Division of Mental Health and Hospitals or the New Jersey Department of Human Services.

Contents

Acknowledgments

In so many ways the successful undertaking of this journey was possible because it was truly a group endeavor. A small nucleus of rather special persons were able, early on, to capture the essence of a collaborative participatory process and so provide the essential direction, leadership, and role modeling. For this we are indebted to Janice Hengle, MS, OTR; Janice McCurdy, ACSW; Charles Mark, PsyD; Natalie Moynihan, MSRN, and Arlene Palasak, MARN. Their creative spirit, professional expertise, courage in risk-taking, and unfaltering commitment to quality care provided the spark and reassurance to others for testing new waters.

To the many many others who came to embrace change and who thus became integral contributing participants and collaborators, we are sincerely grateful. It was this total group effort that made it possible for all of us to be creators of change and to come to know what making a difference is all about.

Gail S. Fidler
Barbara Bristow

Contributor

Suzanne Goren, PhD, RN, has provided consultation to many health care organizations regarding professional practice, service design, and organization development. She co-developed and presented seminars on "Getting Unstuck Without Coming Unglued: Moving from Custodial to Active Treatment," and also has extensive experience in leading workshops and seminars on team building, and management of decentralized systems. In the past, Dr. Goren has held faculty appointments at New York University and the University of Pennsylvania; she is currently Clinical Associate Professor of Nursing at Virginia Commonwealth. She received her masters and doctoral degrees in Nursing from New York University.

Introduction 1

OVERVIEW

The material presented herein is the result of a three-year initiative to transform a state mental health institution from a nursing home care facility to a comprehensive geropsychiatric treatment and rehabilitation hospital focusing on early return to community living. This endeavor involved the generation of fundamental changes in the institution's organization and administrative functions, its clinical policies and practices, its definition of patient needs, intervention strategies, and priorities. These alterations finally brought about significant change in both patient and staff expectations regarding autonomy, achievement, and productivity.

The work described here was carried out from 1985 through 1987. The institution, a 188-bed facility, had for more than eight years been providing long-term nursing care to chronically mentally ill, elderly patients transferred from public psychiatric hospitals. Less than three years after the start of the project, the institution became a fully accredited, certified psychiatric hospital specializing in the active treatment and rehabilitation of New Jersey's mentally ill elderly. Over a three-year period, 133 patients were discharged to community settings in contrast to 21 discharges over the previous three years (1982–1985). Admissions were increased from 78 to 154 with a readmission rate of less than one %. The average length of stay was reduced from 5.2 years to 1.8 years. During the final phase of the project, a state policy change was achieved and 24 patients were directly admitted to the facility from the community for acute, short-term intervention. By 1986 the staff turnover rate had dropped from 21.57%, the highest in the system to the lowest, at a rate of 5.65%.

Our road map for change was planned on the basis of two firmly held tenets. First, the conviction that an environment becomes a therapeutic agent in its own right when its operations and policies and its physical characteristics embody for both patients and staff: a responsiveness to their needs, interests, and concerns; participative problem solving and decision making; an open system of communication; ongoing clarification of roles and interpersonal relationships; purposeful activity; the valuing of personal achievement and contribution; and finally, a comfortable and esthetically pleasing physical environment.

Second, an unfaltering belief that a comprehensive, quality treatment and rehabilitation regimen, focused on maximizing the patient's ability to function as independently as possible, would have positive, productive outcomes for both patients and staff. It was expected that the productive outcomes would be characterized by an increased capacity of the patient to manage the activities of daily living in ways satisfying to themselves and their significant others; a developing sense of competence and positive self-regard on the part of the patient and the staff, a high morale with a commitment to the philosophy and mission of the facility; and, finally, the emergence of a cost-effective operation.

By sharing what we learned and accomplished, it is our hope to add to the knowledge base of the defining and planning of mental health programs for the elderly. It is also our goal to provide a description of the salient characteristics and processes necessary to create a responsive, environment—an environment characterized by on-going role clarification, expectation clarification, and validation of outcomes—an integral part of psychiatric treatment and rehabilitation.

Although exact replication of our model is not the intent of this publication, much of the material is indeed applicable to a variety of settings. There is relevance for day-treatment programs, mental health agencies, nursing homes, and other congregate care settings that serve the cognitively or psychiatrically impaired older adult. In addition, there is much that is applicable to the provision of program services for the chronically mentally ill population.

SERVICE NEEDS

The need for mental health services to the elderly is becoming increasingly evident and urgent. These persons form the fastest growing segment of our population. In the United States, the number of persons over 65 is expected to grow by the year 2000 to about 35 million, an additional 26 million will be added by the year 2020 to 73 million by the year 2080 (Meyers, 1985). It is estimated that approximately 7 million elderly persons currently need some type of mental health assistance (N.J. Dept. of Community Affairs, 1985). In March 1989, the *New York Times* reported that 80% of the elderly who need psychiatric help are not receiving the care they need. The suicide rate among the elderly is the highest of all age groups and approximately 20% of all suicides are committed by people 65 and over. Experts agree that the incidence of mental health problems among older persons is higher than that of the general population (GAO Report, 1982). These current estimates place the incidence of psychiatric problems in the aged population who reside in the community as somewhere between 15% to 25%. For those aged persons in nursing homes, 50% to 70% are reported as exhibiting significant emotional and behavioral problems (N.J. Dept. of Community Affairs, 1985).

Although the need for mental health care among the elderly is more and more evident, statistics indicate a low rate of utilization of services among this group. Nationally, the aged population represents only 2% of the caseloads of private psychiatrists. Less than 1.5% of all expenditures for mental health care in the United States is allocated to community-based services for older persons although they represent more than 11% of the population. The elderly, in spite of need, comprise approximately only 4% of the caseloads of community mental health centers nationally. (GAO Report, 1978) Such under utilization reflects, in part, the reluctance of the elderly to acknowledge their need for help. It also is the result of a priority focus of many community-based mental health programs on vocational training and psychotherapy programs for the young populations. Adding to the emerging crisis, the provision of psychiatric services in nursing homes generally ranges from poor to nonexistent and there are increasing pressures to exclude the mentally ill from these facilities.

As a group, the elderly have unique social, economic, and health needs that mandate separate and different programs. The lifestyle, interests, preferences, and health concerns of this population are indeed dissimilar from other age groups. Frequently there is a diminished social-support system due to the increasing infirmity of the older person and the deaths of relatives and friends. Physical and mental functioning is altered or diminished by the changes and medical problems associated with the aging process. Finally, mobility becomes a challenge and a lack of transportation can be a serious barrier to accessing services and social relationships (GAO Report, 1978). While continuity of services is a significant factor for all populations, it is certainly critical for the elderly. These individuals generally have a lowered tolerance for stress or trauma. Furthermore, diminished resilience makes recovery from illness or injury a slower and, at times, more tenuous process. Thus longer hospital stays, thorough discharge planning, and the provision of well-coordinated aftercare services are essential.

PRIORITIES FOR CHANGE

Our ultimate goal was, of course, to create an active, comprehensive treatment and rehabilitation model. However, the first overall priority was to begin to build an environment that would nurture and support such a goal. The creation of a responsive, clarifying environment that embodied the very principles that characterize adaptive daily living (e.g., independence, collaboration, sharing, positive regard for self and others, purposeful activity) was deemed a most critical first endeavor.

Planning for change involves (a) taking a critical look at the current state of affairs, (b) defining what things will look like when long-range goals are achieved and then on the basis of such data (c) specifying the time-sequenced changes that will need to be made in order to move from point (a) to point (b). Our analysis of the status quo revealed a number of characteristics that would clearly influence the planning and process of change.

One striking asset was the quality of the physical care provided to patients. Medical and nursing care were well above average and patients were well groomed, well dressed, and well fed. This evident concern for and commitment to the health and well-being of the patient was a positive force in the shaping of the new mission.

In the realm of patient program services, several strengths were evident and these provided some critical bridges for transition. An assembly-line workshop offered meaningful activity for those whose values included the work ethic. There was a well-functioning interfaith chaplaincy service and good recreational programs with solid community affiliation and a clearly evident priority of patient satisfaction, comfort, and enjoyment. Social services consistently demonstrated a commitment to family relationships and advocacy for the quality of life for each patient.

On the other side of the coin, there were a number of characteristics that could be expected to present road blocks in the change process. These included:

1. *An Authoritarian Model of Management.* This was a top-down operation. Decisions, problem identifications, and resolutions were all made at the top and handed down to staff. Upward communication was very limited. Management and supervision frequently consisted of written directives and disciplinary codes.

2. *Established Patterns of Dependency.* The patients were dependent on staff and staff were dependent on administration. The parent–child relationship model characterized staff–patient interactions. Being protective of and doing for the patient were valued behaviors. Staff attitudes and actions were frequently infantilizing and expectations for patients' functioning were low. In a similar manner, staff expected management to solve all problems and take responsibility for all decisions. Both patients and staff had learned the helplessness roles.

3. *Lack of Professional Staff and Leadership Roles.* There was a lack of professional direction and leadership as well as insufficient numbers and multidisciplinary breadth of professional staff. Recognition of the value of professional expertise and interdisciplinary contributions were minimal. The clinical leadership vacuum had resulted in limited comprehensive care of patients, role ambiguities, power struggles, and loss of professional pride.

4. *Environmental Barriers.* The physical environment had failed to accommodate the psychological needs and physical limitations of the elderly population. The furniture, colors, light, and sound were poorly used and frequently inappropriate. A lack of congregate space and the arrangement of space diminished patient–staff communication and made socializing and activity areas difficult to create. Accommodations for staff were even more limited. Furnishings and equipment were out of date, inefficient, and unattractive.

5. *Low Staff Morale.* The staff turnover rate was unusually high. Staff projected feelings of anger, powerlessness, ambivalence, and a sense of futility. There was a strong feeling among nursing staff that the quality of care they provided was not appreciated and recognized. There was a decided mistrust of management, fear of reprisal, and an acute sense of vulnerability.

6. *Limited Expectations for Discharge.* Return to the community was not viewed as a viable option for patients. They were not expected to leave and community placements were very limited. The patients and many staff viewed the community as hostile and risky at best.

Thus within the context of this information and the new mission and goals, a long-range plan was designed to move from point (a) to point (b). The main elements of the plan can be summarized as including the following outcome expectations:

- a decentralized, horizontal management system embodying the principles of participative management
- an open communications system
- a total therapeutic community
- an ongoing staff education and development program with a priority focus on team building
- a responsive and attractive physical environment for both patients and staff
- comprehensive interdisciplinary functional-skills assessment of all patients with individual treatment and rehabilitation initiatives based on such assessments
- six functionally homogeneous living units with unit-specific programs
- the creation of a 32-bed, acute, short-term admissions unit to include direct admissions from the community
- collaborative agreements with local community nursing homes and transfer of nursing-home eligible patients to these facilities
- full accreditation from the Joint Commission on Accreditation for Health Organizations (JCAHO) and certification from the Health Care Financial Certification Association (HFCA) as a psychiatric hospital
- development of a coalition with state and local agencies to plan and oversee a community based geropsychiatric day-treatment center, and a housing program for discharged patients as well as for day-treatment center clients.

The transition from a custodial to therapeutic model significantly impacts all aspects of the system. It involves alterations in how staff view the patients and themselves; changes in attitudes, beliefs, and expectations about the "patient role," illness, health, and aging; about self as a therapeutic agent and as a professional. It includes expected change in how patients perceive themselves, their roles, responsibilities, and expectations. This means letting go of the belief that good nursing and good therapeutic care are defined by "doing for" patients and coming to know that supporting and helping patients "do for themselves" is the crux of quality care and treatment. It means reawakening the patients' need for autonomy by supporting and encouraging independence through opportunities and expectations for contribution to self and others.

A therapeutic community and participative management orientation has a far-reaching influence on how an institution is organized, how it operates, defines responsibilities, resolves problems, and reaches decisions. Open communication, an inherent factor in both orientations, is the process for conflict, resolution, and collaborative planning. It enables staff and patients to express opinions, explore alternatives, and arrive at a consensus. Participative management means coming to understand that most problems can be resolved at the level at which they occur and that such resolution most frequently results in productive outcomes and a sense of competence. It requires understanding that the authoritarian model is a one-way communication pattern that encourages dependency among staff and patients, and that the open-systems approach most frequently fosters adult behavior.

A therapeutic community and participative management orientation reflect a respect for the nature and quality of the nonhuman environment. This includes a physical environment that is physically and psychologically safe and barrier free for both patients and staff; one that is responsive insofar as possible to their needs, reflecting a respect for and a valuing of the total institution. It means planning and structuring with patients a living environment in keeping with their cultural norms, age, disabilitiy, and personal preferences. It means effecting a collaborative relationship with staff in the design and operation of their working areas.

Many times, the finest of plans go awry in the implementation phase. In the last analysis, success or failure depends in good measure on the line staff who carry the responsibility and the power to make things happen. Ongoing staff education and development, relevant to the institution's mission and philosophy and to staff interests, competency concerns, and career development, are critical to the quality and efficacy of any endeavor.

Successful treatment and rehabilitation (the function of the system) is a formation of the interaction among patients, staff, and the environment to form an optimum whole system with maximum impact on each part.

In subsequent chapters the most critical components of such a system will be defined and an attempt to describe how they interrelate to form a whole will be made.

REFERENCES

GAO Report. (1978). President's Commission on Mental Health, Task Panel on the Elderly, Government Accounting Office, Washington, D.C.

GAO Report. (September 16, 1982). *The Elderly Remain in Need of Mental Health Services.* Government Accounting Office, Washington, D.C.

Myers, G. C. (1985). Demographics of aging populations—key issues. *Graying Americans and our health system.* Report of the 1985 National Forum on Hospital and Health Affairs. Department of Health Administration, Duke University, Durham, N.C.

New Jersey Department of Community Affairs, Division on Aging. (August 1985). Trenton, New Jersey, *Aging in New Jersey-Sixty-five and older.*

2 Guiding Principles and Philosophy of Patient Care

The importance of having a clearly articulated treatment philosophy or frame of reference cannot be over-emphasized. While a mission statement articulates the purpose of a facility, the philosophic statement establishes the guidelines for how that purpose will be accomplished. It provides the orientation for all patient-care initiatives and treatment plans. The two statements are interrelated. One saying, this is why we exist; the other explaining, this is what we believe and this is the frame of reference with which we will work to achieve our mission.

For example, our mission statement identified the following as the new purpose of the facility; to improve the patient's physical, psychological, and social functioning so that the highest possible level of independence in daily living activities can be achieved; to foster and support individual potential and self-determining behaviors; and, to enable adaptation to community living at a level commensurate with individual capacities, limitations, and needs. In this endeavor, the hospital is committed to operating as a total therapeutic community; to the delivery of a comprehensive continuum of rehabilitation and treatment services; to the development and maintenance of collaborative relationships with community agencies and the public so as to provide a spectrum of community-based service options for patients and enable public understanding and support.

The philosophy of patient care and treatment that was developed relied heavily on the work of Fidler (1984, 1982; Fidler & Fidler, 1978; Fidler & Ridgway, 1955) and was thus based on several assumptions about human performance and the quality of life. These include the belief that achievement of a way of life that sustains health and is more satisfying to self and significant others is measured by the extent of one's success in carrying out, with a relevant degree of autonomy, the fundamental roles and activities of daily living. These encompass (a) the ability to care for and maintain oneself at a level of greater independence than dependence, (b) the ability to be engaged in chosen activities for the sheer personal joy and pleasure in the doing, (c) the ability to contribute to the welfare of others, and (d) the ability to enter into and sustain mutually satisfying interpersonal relationships.

Social efficacy and personal satisfaction relate directly to achieving and maintaining a lifestyle that reflects an age-specific, culturally relevant balance among these roles. Being able to care for one's self at the highest possible level of independence significantly contributes to one's self-regard and sense of being in control. Maintaining a level of independence in self-care and self-maintenance commensurate with one's age, capacities, and limitations has a marked influence on personal satisfaction and the satisfaction of others with whom one lives. It supports personal identity, a sense of competence, integrity, and self-respect.

The ability to pursue personal pleasure, to engage in an activity, to perfect a skill for the sheer enjoyment in the doing (in contrast to pleasing or accommodating others) reinforces a positive self-regard, one's personal value and worth and verifies both the right and the capacity to be self-determining and to value one's own needs, interests, and pursuit of pleasure. Being able to contribute to the welfare of others, to make a discernible contribution to the life of another, to one's family, social group, and/or community verifies social membership and belonging and reaffirms one's social efficacy. Being able to establish and sustain a reciprocal human relationship, to have a friend, to be part of a family, a peer group, to love and be loved are fundamental to the innate human need to be accepted and valued, to experience self as acceptably human. The ability to cope and to manage the expectations of everyday life derive from being able to attain some level of success in each of these roles or sets of behaviors that define human performance. Rehabilitation and treatment initiatives are thus directed toward enabling the patient to achieve an individually appropriate level of independence in each.

The belief system that shaped our treatment and rehabilitation programs as well as the operations of the institution are specifically articulated in a number of principles. We believe these are fundamental to the planning and design of treatment and rehabilitation systems for the elderly.

Principle I: The Attitudes, Values, and Expectations of Staff Significantly Influence the Outcomes of Interventions

It is essential that staff project a belief in the integrity of the individual, a valuing of independence, an expectation that improvement in functioning is attainable and that the quality of life, regardless of age or disability, is indeed important. Researchers are now recognizing that negative staff expectations create the very behavior that they predict in the elderly (Krosberg & Froman, 1975). Another study has shown that when staff are sensitized to the possibilities of improvement in confused older persons, benefits are achieved regardless of the therapeutic approach (Craig & Johnson, 1970). Experience suggests that progress will occur when staff communicate an expectation of improved functioning within an environment that is supportive and respectful of the dignity of both patients and staff. Opportunity for staff to regularly examine and reexamine their attitude and beliefs, and clarify their values is therefore an essential process.

Principles II: The Interrelationship of Mind and Body is an Especially Significant Concept in Designing Services for the Elderly

Medical and psychiatric care must be interrelated as well as comprehensive and take into account the individualized processes of aging. A comprehensive assessment is especially important in the treatment of the geriatric patient because of the complexities that a combination of medical and psychiatric conditions can produce. It is often a challenge to accurately determine the etiology of the symptoms that a patient is manifesting. Medical disorders such as myocardial infarction, urinary tract infection, pneumonia, and cancer may, for example, be evidenced by psychiatric symptoms but remain otherwise hidden. Behavioral symptoms may be a patient's only means of communicating distress related to painful conditions such as arthritis, peptic ulcers, or constipation (Moak, 1988). A loss in functioning should not be routinely accepted as an inevitable part of the aging process. For example, confusion, irritability, depression, and neurologic symptoms are not infrequently related to medication rather than to the aging process per se. A reduction in capacity due to physical and/or mental dysfunction is often remediated in response to appropriate diagnosis and treatment.

Principle III: A Multidisciplinary, Collaborative, Approach is Essential

Assessment and treatment must take into consideration physiologic, psychologic, and performance impairments. A multidisciplinary team approach ensures that the patient is viewed with a wide angle lens that encompasses a number of perspectives and is thus likely to result in treatment initiatives that consider the whole person. Each discipline has a unique contribution to make toward the overall evaluation, goal-setting, treatment-planning, and monitoring processes. It is the special expertise of each discipline that ensures a comprehensive view. The effectiveness of treatment planning is in good measure related to the nature and extent of collaborative exchange, mutual respect, and shared problem solving among all members of the team.

Principle IV: Achievement of the Highest Possible Level of Independent Functioning in Individually Relevant Activities of Daily Living is the Primary Focus of Treatment and Rehabilitation

The purpose of maximizing the ability to perform individually relevant tasks and roles of daily living is so that the individual can achieve and sustain: a positive self-regard, a sense of autonomy, a feeling of having some control over his or her life, and a way of living that is more satisfying than not to self and to one's significant others. The design of services should, therefore, address two interrelated components. These may be broadly categorized as:

1. Services concerned with alleviating or eliminating those physical illnesses or impairments, diseases, mental or psychologic disabilities that interfere with or inhibit the performance of appropriate daily living activities. Activities of daily living that are considered appropriate and important for a given elderly individual depends on that person's characteristic lifestyle and the expectations of that person's living environment. A disability or loss of function carries a different weight or priority of concern in relation to the individual's needs and preferences and the environment's age-specific social and cultural norms of role and task expectations. Individual treatment and rehabilitation goals will have realistic meaning to the degree that they take into account the expectations and the supportive potential of the individual's living environment.
2. Programs that stimulate and support healthy behaviors; those that enable the patient to use, verify, and reinforce individual strengths, abilities, and interests and thus enhance self-regard and the quality of life. Individual skills, interests, and capacities are the bridges to coping skills and adaptive behaviors. A personal sense of competence of being able to achieve derives from doing those things that one does well and which bring a sense of pleasure. Opportunities to use one's skills and abilities in the service of self and others is the essence of motivation and the sense of well-being. Nothing succeeds

like success. It is critical to remember how fragile is the ability to use one's strengths in an institutional setting that limits such opportunities.

Principle V: Independent Functioning of the Elderly is Supported and More Readily Sustained in an Environment that Accommodates their Physical, Sensory, Cognitive, and Perceptual Limitations

Both the physical and interpersonal aspects of the setting must be responsive to physical and psychologic capacities and must be consistently clarified.

The visual, auditory, tactile, and olfactory environments must compensate for sensory losses. The structural components of the environment, the predictability of routines and schedules, consistent time management and other aspects of cognitive cuing are critical for offsetting cognitive limitations of, for example, memory, recall, sequencing, and temporal adaptation. The interpersonal field should consistently and supportively clarify the realities of sight, sound, expectations, achievement, reciprocal caring, and human dignity.

Principle VI: A Sense of Competence, Personal Integrity, and Motivation is Enhanced in an Environment in which Positive Feedback and Verification of Individual Achievement and Contribution are Integral Elements of Administrative, Clinical, and Interpersonal Policies and Behaviors.

Self-esteem, a positive self-regard evolves from evidence of one's strengths and competencies. The intrinsic gratification that follows one's successful testing and clarification of competence is a potent incentive. When significant others (family, authority, peers) acknowledge such effort as having worth and value to the community as a whole, social efficacy and personal worth is confirmed and initiative and motivation is sustained and enhanced (Fidler & Fidler, 1978). Treatment environments for the elderly must always be alert to the significance of positive feedback, supporting and rewarding initiative, and independence and guarding against a focus on disability, or on doing *for* the patient and/or rewarding compliance. By the same token, positive feedback and verification of social efficacy are similarly related to staff motivation, commitment, and productivity.

Principle VII: An Environment that Exemplifies, in Its Daily Operations, the Values of Individual Autonomy, Open Communication, and Collaborative Decision Making, Maximizes the Potential of Patients and Staff.

Opportunities for patients and staff to have choices, to have a say about their treatment or working environments is an essential element in enabling a sense of autonomy, a positive self-regard, high incentive, and productivity. Active participation in such decision making engenders an identity of self as an agent for change, a self capable of influencing events in one's own life, and of being able to make things happen for self and for others.

The need to feel in control of one's life is acknowledged as a universal human need. Studies have indicated that being able to exercise some control over one's environment is critical to physical and psychologic well-being (Teitelman, 1982). On the other hand, a sense of helplessness reduces initiative, assertiveness, motivation, and self-esteem. In a different but related context, management theories have, for many years, affirmed that participative decision making and problem solving between worker and management increased motivation and productivity.

Elderly patients, especially those with the added stress of a psychiatric illness, are particularly vulnerable to helplessness. Chronic mental illness and/or long-term institutionalization frequently create an habitual sedentary lifestyle and exaggerated dependency. Learned helplessness becomes the characteristic of the patient role. In addition, the inability to meet the expectations of daily living, the repeated experiences of failure and loss of autonomy generates a sense of hopelessness, feelings of depression, and/or anger. Intervening and altering such behaviors and expectations requires an environment that is sensitive and responsive to individual differences, one that understands and attends to the psychodynamic, sensory, cognitive, and social-learning aspects of behavior; an environment that provides support, and reassuring expectations for trying out and practicing more independent, self-initiating behaviors; an environment that therapeutically limits risks, ensures success, offers structure and consistency and is characterized by a balance of freedom, control, and incentive tailored to the needs and capacities of the individual patient (Fidler, 1984).

The importance of the patient being actively involved in those choices that impact their lives cannot be overemphasized. It has been demonstrated that the availability of choices, for example, over food, clothing, leisure time, daily activities, not only extends life but significantly enhances the person's sense of satisfaction with that life (Langer & Rodin, 1976; Solomen, 1990). Additionally, staff must be sensitive to the fact that the strangeness of a new environment can be, and frequently is, frightening and confusing. This reality, when coupled with the care-taking, protective behaviors of staff can encourage a sense of vulnerability and helplessness. For many patients, the inability to meet the physical demands of an environment accompanied by the regimentation of a hospital or residential center results in a sense of frustration that may be exhibited by aggression and/or regression. These behaviors then elicit more vigorous custodial or control efforts by the caregivers, which in turn reinforces helplessness and dependency (Levy, 1987).

Open communication and collaborative relationships among staff, between staff and patients, and among patients are important components of a treatment environment. Open communications is the process of operationalizing the concept that patients and staff of all levels have both a responsibility and a right to express opinions, raise questions, make suggestions with the expectations that their ideas and concerns will be heard and respectfully addressed. It is the means of sharing and participating. It is an open dialogue among patients and staff at all levels, with opportunities to resolve issues and problems at their point of origin, argue a point, disagree, make suggestions, all without fear of reprisal. Open communications and shared decision-making processes create and reinforce the awareness that each person, patients and staff, can indeed make a difference; a difference in one's own life and in the lives of others. It provides a model for patients, reassuring and supporting their efforts in working toward more productive self-advocacy, independence, and trusting relationships.

Interpersonal interactions, the design of living and working spaces, and the general tone of the total environment have a significant impact on achieving rehabilitation goals and on patient and staff self-esteem, attitudes, and consequent behaviors.

All persons, patients and staff at all levels have a role, a right, and responsibility to contribute to those decisions that affect their lives as a patient or their role as a staff member. Shared responsibility for the functioning of the institution, for the attainment of its mission, for open communication and participatory decision making creates a *Laboratory for Living* (Fidler & Ridgway, 1955)—an environment for practicing the skills of living, for learning to accommodate the limitation that results from illness or the aging process, and for using one's strengths and skills in creating a more satisfying and productive way of life.

Collaborative working relationships with families and community agencies are essential to helping the patient accomplish the goal of adaptive community living. The hospital is one system in a continuum of systems. Its effectiveness in achieving its mission will depend on the strength of the community liasons it builds.

REFERENCES

Craig, W., & Johnson, J. (1970). Attitude therapy in a crisis intervention program. *Hospital and Community Psychiatry, 21,* 165–168.

Fidler, G. S. (1982). *The lifestyle performance profile: An organizing frame.* In Hemphill, B. (Ed.), *The evaluative process in psychiatric occupational therapy.* Thoroughfare, NJ: Charles B. Slack.

Fidler, G. S. (1984). *The design of rehabilitation services in psychiatric hospital settings.* Laurel, MD: Ramsco.

Fidler, G. S., & Fidler, J. S. (1978). Doing and becoming: purposeful action and self-actualization. *American Journal of Occupational Therapy, 32,* 305–310.

Fidler, G. S. & Ridgway, E. P. (1955). Occupational therapy: Laboratory for living. *Mental Health Views, 3* (3), 66–96.

Krosberg, J., & Froman, J. (1975). Perceptions toward the rehabiitation potential of institutionalized aged. *The Gerontologist, 15,* 403.

Langer, E. J. & Rodin, J. (1976). The effects of choice and enhanced responsibility for the aged. A field experiment in an institutional setting. *Journal of Personality and Social Psychology, 34,* 191–198.

Levy, L. (1987). Psychosocial intervention and dementia, Part 1: State of the art, future directions. *Occupational Therapy in Mental Health,* 7(1), 69–107.

Moak, G. (1988). Treating elderly chronic patients in state hospitals. *Hospital and Community Psychiatry, 39,* 119–124.

Solomon, K. (1990). Learned helplessness in the elderly: Theoretic and clinical considerations. *Occupational Therapy and Mental Health, 10*(3), 31–51.

Teitelman, J. (1982). Eliminating learned helplessness in older rehabilitation patients. *Physical and Occupational Therapy in Geriatrics, 1*(4), 3–10.

3 The Therapeutic Community and Participatory Management

The concept that the total environment of a psychiatric hospital significantly influences treatment has been well supported in the literature for many years. In a related but different context, studies in the fields of management and social psychology have documented the impact of the human environment on worker productivity, job satisfaction, and product quality. It seems reasonable, therefore, to expect that the potential for achieving treatment and rehabilitation goals will be increased to the degree that the total environment exemplifies the focus and inherent expectations of such goals. Rehabilitation and treatment goals reach beyond symptom reduction. They encompass expectations that the patient will achieve some relevant level of self-determination, reciprocal human relationships, meaningful work, and personal need satisfaction. An environment that enables and supports pursuit of these goals in its management and clinical practices is an environment that maximizes the potential for positive outcomes. The creation and maintenance of a clarifying, responsive, total environment becomes a top priority in the treatment and rehabilitation of the older adult.

THE THERAPEUTIC COMMUNITY

In the 19th century, the doctrine of moral treatment revolutionized public institutions for the mentally ill. This philosophy of humane treatment was built on a set of beliefs attesting to the value of caring, human relationships; the importance of a pleasant, friendly environment and the value of daily purposeful activity (Greenblatt, York, & Brown, 1955). It is notable that the decline of this method of patient care seems directly related to the significant social and economic changes that occurred in the mid-to-late 1800s. The increasing rise in the population made it impossible to limit the size of the public mental hospital. At the same time, there was an alarming shortage of psychiatrists and other professionals to service increasing numbers of patients. The large, overcrowded, professionally understaffed public mental institution became a reality. More than a hundred years would pass before the beliefs and concepts of moral treatment were systematically examined and applied to the psychiatric hospital.

In the late 1940s, Harry Stack Sullivan's conceptions of interpersonal relationships significantly extended the dimensions of psychiatric treatment (Sullivan 1947, 1953). His remarkable contributions heightened inquiry into the dynamics of dyadic relationships and broadened the horizons of treatment. Almost simultaneously, treatment of psychiatric casualties during World War II was providing clear evidence of the effectiveness of both group interaction and the setting (Jones, 1962; Wilner, 1981). These developments were the stimulus for bridging the existing gap between theories of psychiatric treatment and social science theories of social adjustment (Wilner, 1958).

The Stanton and Schwartz study of a mental hospital was a landmark in sociopsychiatric inquiry (Stanton & Schwartz, 1934). Its detailed analysis of formal and informal organization, systems of communication, the structure of power, and decision making clearly established that the mental hospital was indeed a social system that shaped the behaviors of both patients and staff. Subsequent research of both public and private hospitals verified the significance of planned and systematic use of the total hospital environment, its physical resources, and its social interactive patterns among all categories of staff and patients (Caudhill, 1985; Greenblatt et al., 1955; Greenblatt, Levinson, & Williams, 1957). Simultaneously, Maxwell Jones' innovative Therapeutic Community provided the model for creating and using a total environment as a method of treatment and rehabilitation (Jones, 1953, 1962, 1976). His formulations became the bench mark for the development and study of a new method of psychiatric treatment that emphasized a democratic social organization, self-determination, group process, and open communication.

During the 1950s and 1960s research produced an exciting and substantive new body of knowledge. Interpersonal relationships; group processes; an open system of communication; decentralized, participatory planning and decision making; purposeful activity; and a responsive, normalized physical environment were identified as critical elements in the operation of a mental hospial and a therapeutic community (Artis, 1962; Cummings & Cummings, 1962; Edelson, 1964; Stainbrook, 1971).

The social and economic changes of the 1970s and 1980s significantly altered the mental health care delivery system. Deinstitutionalization and the priority of community-based treatment has reduced the stature of the public psychiatric hospital, removing it from its previous center stage position. The consequence has been the loss of interest in further examination of the mental hospital as a social system. More serious is the paucity of research in the application of established theories to present day treatment and rehabilitation environments. Although the traditional therapeutic community is best suited for long-term treatment environments, it seems safe to conjecture that many of its elements can be profitably adapted to other settings. An enhanced understanding and appreciation for the therapeutic potential of an interdisciplinary staff, for the rehabilitation potential of the environment, and for patient activities are perhaps the most significant contribution this model has made to the treatment and patient-care system (Gutheil, 1985).

In essence, the therapeutic community is the creation and use of an environment that maximizes collaborative efforts between staff and patients toward achieving the mission and goals of treatment and rehabilitation. It acknowledges that all human relationships and interactions have therapeutic potential for patients and self-actualizing potential for staff. Jones (1976) has referred to it as a cooperative movement within an institution aimed at closing the communication gap between patients and staff for the benefit of all concerned. The model stresses the importance of the total environment, emphasizing its inclusion of relationships among all staff, among patients, between staff and patients, and their engagement in purposeful activities. The environment of a therapeutic community is characterized by:

1. the empowerment of staff and patients through self-determining opportunities, role clarification, and distributive responsibility for the operation of the institution;
2. a democratic social organization that enables collective problem identification, resolution, and distributive responsibility;
3. the use of group process as a primary modus operandi;
4. a system of open communication;
5. meaningful work for both patients and staff;
6. opportunities and responsibilities to engage in those activities that are focused on achieving the goals of treatment and rehabilitation and the mission of the institution;
7. an esthetically pleasing physical environment, which by design and use of living and working spaces is responsive to the needs, role responsibilities, social and cultural norms, and preferences of both patients and staff (Gunderson, 1978; Gutheil, 1985; Karasu, 1984; Stainbrook, 1971).

By promoting self-determination, the therapeutic community helps to counter overdependence. It provides opportunities to learn and practice ways of having an influence on the events in one's life and of being responsible for participation in the community and in one's rehabilitation (Jones, 1953). The shared responsibility and collaborative decision making provides opportunity to practice, in a supportive environment, many skills relevant to community living. The patient is offered responsible, participant involvement in the human relations and administrative decisions that comprise cooperative living. These experiences contribute to the repair of performance skills, to the building of a sense of social adequacy, a positive self-regard, and human relationships. The balance between a focus on socialization and individualization strengthens and supports the productive potential of both staff and patients (Gunderson, 1978; Stainbrook, 1971).

The therapeutic community is a laboratory for social role learning. Social adequacy has been described (Moore & Anderson, 1968) as comprising four major roles or sets of behaviors. (1) The agent role which involves being an agent for self and for others, making things happen, being a cause, and having an influence on the events in one's life; (2) the recipient role which requires being able to appreciate and cope with what one cannot change or influence, accepting the "chanciness" in life events; (3) the significant other role which calls for negotiating and collaborating with others, managing one's own interests and motivations within the context of the needs and interests of others, appreciating the significance of others and managing the give and take of reciprocal engagement; and (4) the evaluator role which involves skills and abilities in making judgments, evaluating and gaining perspective, viewing alternatives and making decisions. Certainly the therapeutic community offers ample opportunities for learning and practice in each of these roles.

One important tenet of the therapeutic community is that staff and patients must feel that they are engaged in constructive and meaningful work. Their activities must make a difference and they need to see the result of their work. Thus, staff must have evidence that they are indeed involved in defining, clarifying, and carrying out the mission of that institution.

Patients must be active participants in planning, carrying out, and evaluating their treatment and rehabilitation.

A system of open communication is integral to the functioning of a therapeutic community. Lines of communication must ensure that information sharing, the exchange of ideas and opinions and other interpersonal interaction flow upward, downward, and horizontally. The daily therapeutic community meeting is fundamental to these processes. Jones (1953) has described this event as a daily meeting of all patients and staff to examine the day-to-day problems of patients and the living unit. These group encounters focus on discussing and resolving the general problems involving human relations and administrative policies that stem from living in a collective society. This process is one of the best insurances against too great a gap between therapeutically desirable operations of a unit and its actual functioning (Stainbrook, 1971). Consistency is an essential ingredient. The time or place of the meeting should not be changed except in emergencies or after a consensus has been reached among the members. Furthermore it must be clear that each staff assigned to the unit is expected to attend. This expectation should include those housekeeping and/or maintenance staff who are regularly on the floor. Circle seating facilities exchange among members and provides a more democratic mix of patients and staff. There is an advantage to having the meeting held in a visible place near the center of patient activity. Patients who are reluctant to attend or for whom attention span is a problem, can observe and/or join for brief periods until they are able to participate more fully.

Frequently staff and patients will ask what is appropriate content for the therapeutic community meeting? Is this group therapy? How is it different? Ultimately, these questions get sorted out over a period of time as staff and patients build norms and establish trust. The question is best addressed by reiterating and clarifying the purpose and the focus of the therapeutic community meeting. In essence, the goal of these meetings is to create a living environment that will maximize potential for accomplishing individual goals as a participant in the institution. In this context, content will most frequently relate to cooperative planning of activities, feedback from staff and patients regarding activities and routines, unit morale and interpersonal/group tensions, administrative policies and decisions, physical environment issues, and the general sharing of information. The frame of reference for exploring and addressing issues will depend on the institution's philosophy and certainly on the professional sophistication and training of the staff. A post meeting is held by staff immediately after the community meeting. The purpose is to review and examine what has gone on in the community meeting. This critique includes, for example, the nature of staff and patient participation, the tone of the meeting and of the unit, a critique of the group process, identification and discussion of any stress signal from the patients, and the nature of staff teamwork.

The goals of the therapeutic community can best be achieved when a hospital is organized into small, decentralized units. These small units help to facilitate face-to-face communication and foster a sense of identity and belonging. The institution's organizational structure and style of management must support and reflect the values of the therapeutic community. Conveying the feeling of hope is one of the most subtle but most significant aspects of the management of the therapeutic milieu (Stainbrook, 1971). The way in which an institution is organized, its administrative policies and procedures, and its style of operating set a tone of expectations for staff and patient behaviors (Bell & Ryan, 1985; Islam & Turner, 1982).

PARTICIPATORY MANAGEMENT

It is interesting to note that the business world has in recent years evidenced a renewed focus on the importance of the environment and of people. Current literature in management (Bennis & Nanus, 1985; Bolman & Deal, 1984; Kantor, 1983; Peters & Watterman, 1982) describes the most successful companies as those whose management practices include strong human resource components. Those whose operations are guided by concepts of productivity through people, through worker participation and involvement.

The historically significant Hawthorn study and the related research of Mayo during the 1920s and 1930s demonstrated that human relationships were a critical force in worker productivity (Mayo, 1933). The ensuing human-relations movement in industry markedly altered management theories and placed a high priority on group process and interpersonal dynamics in management training and practice (Homan, 1950). More recently, the impressive success of the Japanese and the pressures of world-market competition has generated a reawakening of the human aspects of management and operations, emphasizing worker participation in decision making and planning (Yates, 1985).

Participatory management is based on the belief that any complex organization is best managed on a decentralized basis; that most problems can be resolved at the level of their occurrence; that the role of management is to provide an environment in which staff feel valued and can see the results of their influence and contributions; that given appropriate opportunities, people will function at a responsible level and that the small working group is the most successful process for achieving participation, enabling a sense of being part of the whole and being engaged in meaningful work. Finally, that the group-process method tends to result in more options, provides immediate feedback, overcomes resistance to change, and addresses the need of individuals to feel a part of the larger whole (Shaskin, 1982).

Management theories and studies support the belief that when operational models encompass participative planning and decision making among staff, when there is a discernible valuing of interpersonal relationships and individual effort, a sense of ownership and commitment to the organization emerges. There is high productivity and end-product quality (Beck & Hillmar, 1986; Bennis, 1976; Hersey & Blanchard, 1982; Merkel & Pollard, 1987).

The characteristics of a participatory model of management can be summarized as follows:

Organizational Values: Participatory management principles are expressed as part of the organization's value system and operationalized within the organization.

Role Clarification: There is ongoing definition of each individual's contribution to the organization and to the work group, a continuing clarification of what is mine, yours, and ours; and how one can best work together to achieve mutual goals.

Supportive Environment: Management creates an environment in which there is freedom and trust to express opinions, state issues, and concerns without fear of reprisal; communication is open and direct. Management is committed to supplying the necessary resources to accomplish the goals of the organization.

Empowerment/Self Worth: Employees are involved in decision-making processes and are encouraged to use their skills and competencies to build a working group that makes high quality decisions and thus enables a sense of competence, achievement, and pride.

Participative Teamwork: The small working group is the principle method for operationalizing the participatory model of management and accomplishing the goals of the organization.

SIMILARITY OF MODELS

It becomes evident that the therapeutic community and participative management have much in common. Both strive for open communication wherein issues, problems, and ideas can be discussed and argued without retribution. The two models enable and support participative planning and decission making through decentralization and the use of the small working group. Each clearly acknowledges the importance of role clarification and recognition of individual needs and competencies. Both models consider the commitment and active support of top management to be an absolute essential.

Perhaps the most significant contribution of each is in their responsiveness to the need for performance satisfaction. These models address the human need to be engaged in meaningful activities, recognizing that meaningless work alienates people from both the process and the product. Achieving a sense of accomplishment by seeing a task through to completion is an inherent construct of each. The cornerstone of the therapeutic community and participative management is empowerment and self-determination, through engagement in decision making. The universal human need for autonomy and a sense of control over one's life is verified and given credibility. The need to affiliate, to be part of a group and engaged in reciprocal relationships is addressed by the group context that is fundamental to both models.

By responding to these basic human needs, the therapeutic community and participatory management are vehicles for achieving the highest possible levels of performance and actualizing the potential of each participant—patient and staff.

Kramer and Kramer (1976) have compared a therapeutic model with what they describe as a custodial model. The custodial model, they suggest, is the more traditional bureaucratic style of institutional management. This model incorporates characteristics that encourage dependency and regressive behavior on the part of both staff and patients. It is patient role and disability focused, it encourages typical parent–child patterns of relationship, limits upward communication, and is repressive. Conflict is hidden and content is often more important than process. Operations are authoritarian and efficient and when there is upset, it is likely to be expressed symbolically rather than directly. Things are not what they seem. By contrast, the therapeutic community model is characterized by open communication, saying what one thinks, by democratic, collaborative processes that are time-consuming and ripe with argument and debating. Conflicts are out in the open and process is often more important than content. There is a typical adult to adult pattern of relationships with encouragement for independence and collaborative efforts. Things are what they seem.

In many ways communication is the core of a "community" model. A system of open communication is indispensable for the successful functioning of a therapeutic community and/or a participatory management model. Open communication means an environment and process that supports and makes it possible for members of the community (staff and patients) to say what they think. It means freedom to raise questions, express opinions, argue a point, explore issues, criticize, express anger, all without fear of reprisal. Reducing and eliminating the fear of what will happen "when I speak my mind" requires the firm commitment of management to free and open expression. It requires the initial courage of a few staff who are willing to take a risk and thus make it possible for others to see that saying what one thinks is safe and acceptable. It involves accepting that such change does indeed take time. Time for a sense of trust to develop out of the demonstrated commitment of both management and staff to honor the freedom to express an opinion.

When there is open communication the influence of rumor and hearsay is diminished. What is going on and what is being planned is no longer a secret because there is ongoing exchange of information, an airing of ideas, issues, and conflicts. In a therapeutic community, conflict, disagreement, and problems do not disappear. What does change is that they are out in the open where they can be examined and worked through. In fact, in a well-functioning community there are frequent heated arguments; noisy, direct confrontations. There is far less silent resistance, quiet frustration, or complaining. The result is increasing awareness that one can make a difference by speaking up, and that doing so does *not* result in reprisal but rather clarifies issues, leads to wiser decisions, builds trust, and strengthens relationships. In such an environment there is a growing sense of personal value, a respect for self and others. Furthermore, open communication among staff as we have stated earlier, provides a model for patients, reassuring and supporting their efforts in working toward more adult self advocacy, independence, and trusting relationships.

Closely related and in many ways an inherent part of open

communication is the participatory decision-making process. Collaborative decision making means that all persons, patients and staff, at all levels have a part in the decision-making process. Each has a role, a right, and a responsibility to contribute to the formulation of those decisions that significantly affect their life as a patient or their functioning as a member of the staff. From personal experiences each of us has learned that expressing our opinions, having input into a decision, does not always mean that the decision we want will be the one that prevails. Sometimes we win, sometimes we lose, and, more frequently than not, there is a mixture of both in compromise. It works the same way in a therapeutic community!

Collaborative or shared decision making is the way that staff participates in the operation and management of the institution. In such a process one of the first questions is who should be involved in which decisions? There are a few ground rules that can help in beginning to sort out a response to this question. Generally speaking, an individual should be involved in those decisions that significantly affect their working role and functions or their patient roles and living, those that significantly affect daily life at the institution, those about which they have first hand knowledge or expertise, those which they are expected to carry out and finally, those which impact their human rights and responsibilities.

Another dimension of collaborative decision making concerns "the what and the who of collaboration." This involves addressing questions such as:

Which decisions can I make on my own without necessarily consulting anyone? Generally speaking, one is free to make a decision without consulting others when the results of that decision have little or no impact on anyone else. The obvious exception, of course, is an acute emergency when one may need to take immediate autonomous action.

What decisions must I make in collaboration with others, and, furthermore, which decision with whom? In essence, which decisions affect which persons and groups, and therefore, with whom must I share decisions and about what? In deciding who must share in the decision making, the question is who is affected? Is it limited to the floor and only those who work on that floor? If so, then it probably need not go beyond those staff and patients. Does it impact the total unit? the total institution? Would the decision alter a policy, a standard, and at what level? Does the decision require special knowledge or expertise? These are some of the questions that help to define who makes which decisions.

Which decisions are beyond my control, influence, or expertise? In a large society or bureaucracy there are many policies, regulations, laws, etc. that affect us but over which we have very limited, if any, direct control. "Where one sits," that is the status, power, or nature of one's position frequently determines the degree of one's decision-making influence. For example, a state legislator is significantly involved in making laws and related decisions. A voter has some, but not equal, influence. Similarly, line staff usually has limited or no input into many decisions of the top bureaucracy. Civil Service regulations, health care standards, state and federal regulations are a few such examples. Then there are decisions that require special knowledge such as a medical diagnosis, family therapy issues, psychologic evaluations and the like. Knowing and understanding the limit of one's influence or expertise is critical for avoiding frustration or failure.

Obviously, the more persons involved in an organization and the difference among these persons, the more complex the decision-making process. Thus the continuing questions of what is *my* responsibility, what is *ours,* who makes up the "ours" and what is beyond our or my scope of influence or knowledge? Attempts to eliminate or reduce the questions too frequently result in autocratic and expedient rules. Line staff makes rules for patients, supervisors make rules for lower line staff, managers make rules for supervisors, the C.E.O. makes rules for managers, and so on. The result, of course, is a sense of frustration, futility, and powerlessness on the part of everyone. The creation of clearly structured "groupings" or forums for communication and decision making at all levels helps to sort out who decides what with whom, as well as clarifying the procedure for appropriate decision making and problem resolution. An example of such a structure is depicted in the communication loop, Figure 3.1, on p. 39.

The administrative structure and functioning of an organization, its group and interpersonal relationships, and its physical environment are elements of a dynamic interactive system that shapes and defines the nature, quality, and outcomes of patient treatment and rehabilitation. The planning and management of these elements is every bit as important as the planning and management of treatment, per se.

EXAMPLES OF APPLICATION

The translation of these constructs into practice required some major organizational and administrative changes within the institution. The first step was to acknowledge that changes in the structure and operations of the institution, in the development of an interdisciplinary professional staff, and the education of staff and patients needed to be planned and be well into the implementation phase before any major change could begin in the structure and content of patient programs and services. Congruence among administrative philosophy and procedures, staff attitudes and roles, and the content and processes of patient treatment was deemed essential.

Changes in the structural operations of the institution and staff development were planned and implemented simultaneously. The principal focus was to create an organizational structure and management process that would facilitate shared, collaborative decision making, stimulate and support open communication, and generate a commitment and sense of ownership regarding the institution's new mission. To this end, the first initiative was to strengthen and empower each professional discipline by recruiting qualified staff; appointing full-time department heads; clarifying roles, responsibilities, and expertise; and giving each department the authority to manage the operations of their discipline. A qualified clinical director was recruited to provide the overall clinical leadership and stimulate the development of professional leadership and collaborative potential within and among disciplines. Our endeavor to empower the clinical and rehabilitation disciplines and strengthen professional expertise can be viewed as being in conflict with the democratic principles of the therapeutic community. However, this initiative was based on the firm belief that there is a direct relationship between the quality of patient services and the number and quality of professional staff. Furthermore, experience has demonstrated that true, democratic, interdisciplinary collaboration is far more possible when each discipline can take pride in and respect the quality of its unique service. Under such circumstances of equality, defensiveness is reduced and the capacity for respecting and hearing others is enhanced.

Simultaneously, the executive staff was fully oriented to the concepts and operating procedures of participatory management and the therapeutic community models. All standing committees of the institution were reviewed and revised to clarify roles and responsibilities, establish lines of communication and accountability, define and emphasize interrelationships. All committees were housed in either the clinical/medical committee or the support services committee. The executive committee included the top management of each Clinical and Support department. These revisions created a structure for collaborative endeavor and horizontal communication. Procedures for establishing the goals and objectives of the institution and allocating resources were revised to provide for participation of staff at all levels. Each department and each patient living unit was given responsibility for developing their yearly goals and objectives and related budget requests. The preparation of a comprehensive budget request and set of goals for the institution as a whole involved dialogue and decisions among departments within either the clinical/medical or support services committee. When these groups reached consensus their recommendations were presented to the executive committee for final approval. Because all members of this committee had participated in one or more phases of the development process, this last step was typically free of problems. Staff ownership of the final product was clear. Reaching consensus on these matters and other management issues required ongoing dialogue, negotiation, and compromise among all groups at all levels until consensus was reached.

Initially, these procedures were very stressful for staff as they challenged many traditional beliefs and values. The awareness that it was far less risky and more expedient when management was autocratic was both an overt and covert force in almost all aspects of operations at all levels for quite some time. Ultimately, the rewards of making a difference, of having some control over events, the sense of group belongingness, and ownership became sufficient incentive to continue to work at perfecting the process of participatory decision making.

To further bridge the communication gap between staff and management, copies of the minutes of each of the three major management committees (executive, clinical/medical, and support services) were sent to all departments and to each of the seven patient living units. These copies were kept in a notebook in the central area of each department and patient living unit. Patients and staff were encouraged to read these, critique and discuss issues during regular floor and community meetings and give feedback to the committees.

An open, all hospital staff community meeting was initiated and held on a monthly basis. This forum was intended to provide an opportunity for line staff to meet and communicate with the chief executive officer and the executive management staff. The meeting was informal in that no agenda was prepared and staff were free to raise any issue or make any comment they wished. All executive and management staff were expected to attend and participate in a facilitative role. All employees of the institution were encouraged to attend and adjustments in work schedules were arranged to enable maximum participation and to include as many evening staff as possible. A second meeting on the same day was held with the evening and the night staff. These night meetings were one of a number of initiatives aimed at mainstreaming evening and night staff. The standard "9 to 5" orientation and the disassociation of evening and night staff so characteristic of professional staff began to change as late afternoon and evening team meetings, night case conferences, family counseling, and teaching seminars became a regular part of operations.

At the beginning of the large, open community meetings, all staff were extremely wary. Top management felt vulnerable and argued against the idea. Line staff were suspicious and withholding. Similarly there was an air of discomfort and strangeness among clinical and support services personnel. Staff's orientation to authority and management was evident in a consistent pattern of directing all comments and questions to the chief executive officer, seldom to other management staff and never to one another. Issues were raised in a way that clearly reflected staff's expectation that management's role was to resolve problems. Their response to being encouraged to resolve an issue among themselves was one of anger and distrust with accusations about management not caring. Understandably, only as they were able, over time, to see and know that management was sincere about empowering staff and supporting shared decision making, were they able to begin to take responsibility. It was at least a year before this meeting represented a true dialogue and staff were able to openly discuss, argue, and reach closure among themselves with only marginal attention to the chief executive officer. Attendance, over time, increased significantly with a majority of staff regularly and actively involved.

As a way of improving communication the clinical staff established *The Morning Meeting.* This meeting was held at the beginning of each day to provide feedback concerning events, issues, and concerns that had emerged within the patient living units during the previous evening and night. It was also a time for review of the pending day's schedules, patient appointments, need for special consultations, patients in crisis, and so on. These meetings were attended by a significant representation from all disciplines as well as clinical and medical administration. They were a daily forum for the exchange of information for identification of emergent issues, and clarification of how these would be addressed.

Efforts were begun to strengthen and empower the Patient Council and reduce the "hand holding" by staff. Independent leadership was supported and the group was encouraged to broaden their focus and areas of concern. However, progress was slow. The dependency-promoting effects of institutional life, an environment that had not expected them to be self-reliant or responsible had taken its toll. The patients' integration of these expectations were being reinforced by staff's helping and "caring for" behaviors in all realms of the patients' lives. It was evident that change would come slowly and only as the total environment could nurture and expect self-reliance and a sense of responsibility.

Daily therapeutic community meetings were initiated on each patient living unit and the training of selected staff to function as group facilitators was begun. The role of facilitator was emphasized throughout the training in order to counter typical expectations that being designated a leader meant being in charge, and being responsible for what happened in the group. By contrast, the focus was on learning and practicing ways of helping others express ideas and opinions, ways of facilitating a give-and-take dialogue, of helping the group handle conflict and give feedback in a helpful way. Skills of observation, listening and reflecting, techniques for enabling problem identification, clarification and resolution were examined, practiced, critiqued, and repracticed.

A comprehensive staff education plan was formulated with a first priority on team building, and thus on those processes that enable an aggregate to become a collaborative, productive working group. A fundamental belief of the participatory management model is that problems are best resolved at the level of their occurrence. Resolutions made at this level are owned by staff and will more readily be sustained. However, shared decision making will work only in relationship to staff's comfort with and skill in collaborative processes. Participatory decision making breaks with the traditional way in which both management and line staff have always viewed responsibility for decisions. What becomes evident is that staff is as reluctant to take responsibility as management is to relinquish authority. It is less risky to blame others than to take responsibility. Autocratic decision making is not as frightening as a responsibility for collective decisions. There was ongoing reluctance and related problems whether the issues were treatment planning, floor management, or allocation of resources. Staff education and training thus had as its first mission the learning and practice in collective problem solving, group process, and interpersonal relationships as these related to the business of participatory decision making.

Finally, a long range plan was developed to refurbish and remodel the physical environment of the institution. The first priority of this endeavor was to improve the quality of patient living and staff working areas. This decision was based on the conviction that the physical environment is a force that shapes staff and patient morale and productivity. Thus the incentive was to create an environment that was comfortable, efficient, and attractive; one that would reflect a positive self-regard and a positive regard for the institution and its mission.

Creating an environment that exemplifies the principles of participatory management and the therapeutic community means creating a total structure and process of open communication, collaborative engagement and decision making. Figure 3.1 delineates the structure and procedures of our decision making and communication processes.

As shown in this diagram, there were two all-hospital forums, the Patient Council and the Staff Open Community Meeting. These forums, in addition to their defined purpose, served in many ways as a safeguard against issues getting lost at any level in the system. Because these forums included all patients and all staff, there was little likelihood of any significant issue falling through the cracks. They were indeed monitors of concerns and issues moving through the system in a timely fashion. In addition, the business of the institution was carried out by seven small units or working groups. Each had the responsibility for managing a special area of concern, for generating the necessary dialogue and information sharing to sustain a productive community and each had the authority to manage their charge. The prinicple focus of each forum and working group is summarized as follows:

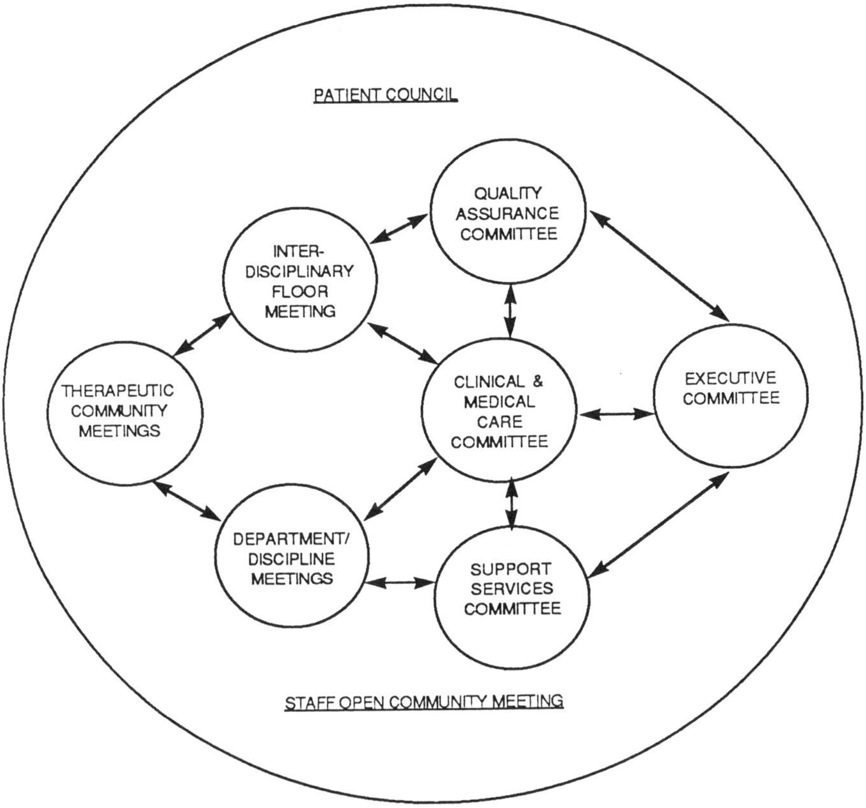

Figure 3.1 Communication loop

The Patient Council was one formal structure and process for patients to deal with those matters that had an impact on their general welfare, comfort, treatment, rehabilitation, and quality of life. It included all patients and was a monthly forum for sharing ideas, generating special projects, discussing issues, resolving problems and/or referring these as necessary to appropriate others as indicated in Figure 3.1.

The Staff Open Community Meeting was a monthly all-staff forum for raising and clarifying issues, expressing opinions, airing differences, exchanging and sharing information. It provided opportunity for staff to get to know others throughout the institution and to communicate, face-to-face with management. Issues and/or recommendations raised at this meeting were immediately directed to the appropriate person or group for action.

The Therapeutic Community Meetings were the hub of patient–staff communication and collaboration. Meetings occurred daily on each floor for the purpose of discussing and dealing with concerns, daily events, and issues related to any aspect of life on the floor. Any problem that emerged and could not be resolved at this level because it required communication and negotiation with others, was presented by a designated community member to appropriate others for mutual resolution.

The Interdisciplinary Floor Meetings were biweekly interdisciplinary forums that were held on each floor and included all staff working on that floor. These meetings were concerned with the management and coordination of patient care and treatment, and with the milieu on the floor for the purpose of maximizing services to the patients and enhancing staff sharing, and collaborative decision making. Issues that extended beyond the scope of the floor were communicated and referred to the appropriate person or committee for mutual resolution. The clinical administrator was responsible for providing ongoing feedback to and from the Clinical/Medical Care Committee.

The Department/Discipline Meetings were biweekly meetings concerned with the operations of a department or discipline, its roles and functions, relationships with other departments and services, staff supervision and education, quality assurance and standards, program planning, and evaluation. Department heads provided feedback, resolved issues, and referred other issues to their appropriate body, either Clinical/Medical Care or Support Services committees.

The Clinical/Medical Care Committee carried overall responsibility for the direction, management, and coordination of all patient treatment and rehabilitation programs and services. This committee represented the top clinical/medical authority, formulating patient care and treatment policies and procedures. Membership included each clinical/medical department head and the director of quality assurance. Feedback to and from the patient council, therapeutic community meetings, departmental meetings, and interdisciplinary floor meetings comprised essential business of this committee.

The Support Services Committee was responsible for the overall management and coordination of the policies and procedures of engineering and maintenance services, food service, business and finance, housekeeping, fire and safety, and laundry. Membership on this committee included the department heads of each of these services.

The Quality Assurance Committee held responsibility for the overall development and monitoring of quality assurance policies, procedures, and programs.

The Executive Committee was the executive arm of the Clinical/Medical Care and the Support Services committees. This committee gave final approval to all policies and procedures of the institution, was responsible for overseeing all operations of the facility and was the official link between the institution and external agencies and bodies. Membership included the Chief Executive Officer, the Clinical and Medical Directors, the Hospital Administrators for Clinical Services and for Support Services, the Director of Quality Assurance and the Director of Personnel.

This total system operated on the principle that problems are best understood and resolved at the level of their occurrence, that productive decisions are the result of a well-informed group working collaboratively and democratically to define the issues, clarify roles, and reach resolutions.

REFERENCES

Artis, K. L. (1962). *Milieu therapy in schizophrenia,* New York: Grune and Stratton.

Beck, A. C., & Hillmar, E. D. (1986). *Positive management practices,* San Francisco: Jossey-Bass.

Bell, M. D., & Ryan, E. R. (1985). Where can therapeutic communities ideals be recognized? An examination of three environments. *Hospital and Community Psychiatry, 36,* 1286–1290.

Bennis, W. G., & Nanus, B. (1985). *Leaders: A strategy for taking charge.* New York: Harper & Row.

Bennis, W. G., Benne, K., & Chin, R. (Eds.). (1976). *The planning of change,* 3rd Ed. New York: Reinholt and Winston.

Bolman, L. G., & Deal, T. E. (1984). *Modern approaches to understanding and managing organizations.* San Francisco: Jossey-Bass.

Caudhill, W. (1958). *The psychiatric hospital as a small society.* Cambridge: Harvard University Press.

Cummings, J., & Cummings, E. (1962). *Ego and milieu.* New York: Atherton Press.

Edelson, M. (1964). *Ego psychology, group dynamics, and The therapeutic community.* New York: Grune and Stratton.

Greenblatt, M., York, R. H., & Brown, E. L. (1955). *From custodial to therapeutic patient care in mental hospitals.* New York: Russell Sage Foundation.

Greenblatt, M., Levinson, D. J., & Williams, R. H. (1957). *The patient and the mental hospital.* Glencoe, IL: Free Press.

Gunderson, J. G. (1978). Defining the threapeutic processes in psychiatric milieus. *Psychiatry, 41,* 327–335.

Gutheil, M. (1985). The therapeutic milieu: Changing themes and theories. *Hospital and Community Psychiatry, 36,* 1279–1285.

Hersey, P., & Blanchard, K. (1982). *Management of organizational behavior,* 4th ed. Englewood Cliffs, NJ: Prentice Hall.

Homan, G. C. (1950). *The human group.* New York: Harcourt, Brace.

Islam, A., & Turner, D. L. (1982). The therapeutic community: A critical reappraisal. *Hospital and Community Psychiatry, 33,* 651–653.

Jones, M. (1953). *The therapeutic community.* New York: Basic Books.

Jones, M. (1962). *Social psychiatry.* Springfield, IL: Charles C Thomas.

Jones, M. (1976). *Maturation of the therapeutic community: An organic approach to health and mental health.* New York: Human Sciences.

Kantor, R. (1983). *The change makers.* New York: Simon & Shuster.

Karasu, T. B. (1984). *The psychiatric therapies.* Washington, DC: American Psychiatric Press.

Kramer, C. H., & Kramer, J. R. (1976). *Developing a therapeutic community.* Springfield, IL: Charles C Thomas.

Mayo, E. (1933). *The human problems of an industrial civilization.* New York: MacMillan.

Merkel, W. T., & Pollard, C. A. (1987). Applying modern management principles to clinical administration of a behaviorally oriented in-patient unit. *Hospital and Community Psychiatry, 38,* 152–159.

Moore, O. K., & Anderson, A. R. (1968). *Some principles for clarifying educational environments.* University of Pittsburgh: Research and Development Center.

Peters, T. J., & Watterman, R. H., Jr. (1982). *In search of excellence: Lessons from America's best run companies.* New York: Harper & Row.

Shaskin, (1982). *A manager's guide to participative management.* College Park, MD: American Management Associations.

Stainbrook, E. (1971). The hospital as a therapeutic community. In Freedman, A. (Ed.), *Treating mental illness: Aspects of modern therapy.* New York: Anthenium Press.

Stanton, A. H., & Schwartz, M. S. (1934). *The mental hospital.* New York: Basic Books.

Sullivan, H. S. (1947). *Conceptions of modern psychiatry.* Washington, DC: William Alanson White Psychiatric Foundation.

Sullivan, H. S. (1953). *The interpersonal theory of psychiatry.* New York: Norton.

Wilner, H. A. (1958). *Social psychiatry in action: A therapeutic community.* Springfield, IL: Charles C Thomas.

Wilner, H. A. (1981). Defining and understanding the therapeutic community. *Hospital and Community Psychiatry, 32,* 95–99.

Yates, D. (1985). *The politics of management.* San Francisco: Jossey-Bass.

4 The Nonhuman Environment: Its Meaning and Uses

Studies concerning the significance of the physical environment of an institution have lagged far behind those related to the interpersonal field. Although the effect of a hospital environment was emphasized as early as 1860 by Florence Nightingale, there is a relative paucity of information regarding this aspect of health care delivery. The total environment or milieu that comprises a hospital, an institution, or agency can be defined as is the proverbial coin, by its two sides. Each distinguishable but fused to form the whole. One part of an institution's milieu includes its interpersonal structures, procedures, and relationships; the human aspects of operations. The other dimension embodies the physical qualities: architectural design and structure, its schedules, routines, and habits that are the nonhuman aspects of operations. Each is characteristically different but necessarily integrated to form the total character and meaning of the institution.

The nonhuman environment is indeed a significant force. It symbolizes the attitudes, values, and beliefs that characterize an institution. It is an agent in its own right for either productive or counterproductive activity. Finally, it offers a rich potential for reinforcing and supporting the mission of an institution and the healthy capacities of the patient.

SHAPING PERSPECTIVES AND ATTITUDES

Buildings, through their design, use of space, light, color, and furnishings have many symbolic meanings. The physical environment of the entrance and the total space of a corporate headquarters building, for example, sends a clear message about how that enterprise regards itself, its mission, and its clients. The distinction between the private sector and the public or state-operated hospital, for instance, is usually striking. The most frequent explanations for the apparent disregard of the public hospital for its physical environment is the lack of funds and the importance of not using taxpayers' money for the luxuries of attractiveness and beauty. Such an explanation is greatly weakened by the reality that attractiveness and comfort are not necessarily costly. Much beauty and attractiveness can be achieved at very little cost.

One can conjecture that the typically drab and/or sterile atmosphere of many public institutions reflects an institution's regard for its mission, its staff, and the people it serves. Wolfensberger (1972, p. 57) makes the point quite well, stating: "Human services are generally rendered inside of buildings, and these buildings often affect the way these services are or can be rendered, how they are perceived by the public, how the public perceives the recipients of these services, and how the recipients perceive themselves." Thus not only does the physical environment reflect how the public views the institution and its mission, it also symbolizes and reflects how the roles and functions of staff and patients are viewed by themselves and others. How staff is expected to perform and patients to behave are manifested in the structure and order of the physical environment. The environment does indeed speak louder than words in many instances.

There is increasing evidence that the nonhuman environment influences the delivery of services and the outcome of services. An attractive, comfortable environment, one that supports the well-being and productive needs of staff and patients projects a positive regard for self, for others and their mission. Simultaneously, such an environment engenders feelings of pride and self-value and motivates productivity (Kiernat 1985; Kramer & Kramer, 1976; Wolfensberger 1972).

Hospitals with extended stay policies, long-term care facilities, and nursing homes are examples of what may be termed total institutions. As such they pose a possible threat to the autonomy and individuality of the patient or resident. Goffman (1961) describes total institutions as closed worlds in which the normal barriers separating sleep, recreation, and work are eliminated. He defines the four major characteristics of such environments as including: (1) all aspects of living occur in the same place and under the same authority; (2) each phase of the daily activity is carried on in the company of others, all of whom are treated alike and required to do the same things; (3) all daily activities are tightly scheduled and imposed by rulings from above; and (4) the mandated activities and schedules are purportedly designed to fulfill the official aims of the institution. It is not difficult to see how a person's individuality and personal lifestyle become at risk under such circumstances. It would seem equally obvious that the design and use of environments to counter and guard against such deindividuation should be a critical aspect of organizational management.

Accreditation and certification agencies have had a significant impact on improving the physical environment of hospitals, nursing homes, and other health care facilities. The right to privacy, to have and keep secure one's personal possessions, to have easy access to a telephone, to send and receive uncensored mail are all required by standards and accreditation regulations. There are, however, other important concerns that are less explicitly addressed by standards and regulations. The first of these relates to the opportunities the environment affords for making choices. Having options, being able to choose from among several alternatives is acknowledged as a significant component in determing the level of one's life satisfaction. As aging changes one's lifestyle, alternatives become more limited and the opportunity for choice more valued. A responsive, health-sustaining environment provides for and ensures a variety of choices relative to daily living activities, social relationships, room decor, dress and the like. When the environment encourages and supports individual freedom to make choices, the sense of being in control of the important aspects of one's life is sustained and one's personal identity is affirmed (Langer & Rodin, 1976; Maier & Seligman, 1976).

The extent to which the environment encourages and permits choices reflects how the patient or resident of the facility is viewed. Role perceptions, that is, what behaviors are expected of the patient and of staff, are evident in an institution's environmental characteristics and designs. By the same token, what is reflected or symbolized in such structures, elicits and reinforces the expected behaviors. The accessibility of staff; the absence of isolating or protective partitions; staff offices on the floors of the patient living units; accessible switches and dials for lights, televisions, and radios; face-to-face dialogue in preference to written communiques and directives; esthetically pleasing, user-friendly patient and staff living and working areas are all clear statements of the valuing and respect for both patient and staff. Such messages have an impact on attitudes and behaviors as well as being a potent public-relations medium. This became quite evident as our redecorating and refurbishing projects were being completed. Staff and patients expressed a new sense of pride and caring concern for their living and working areas. One staff member who had been especially critical of the proposed improvements, charging that they were a waste of time and money and would only be ruined by the carelessness of patients and staff, came to a different conclusion some months later. "I was wrong," she declared, "it's a joy to come to work, to walk into this building, it makes me proud to be here." Similarly, visitors regularly commented about the attractiveness of the total facility, expressing a sense of wonder that it was a state institution. It was evident that we were being seen in a new light.

How the institutionalized elderly are viewed is reflected in many aspects of institutional environments. The perception that these persons are more childlike than adult, as well as being "not quite with it," gets played out in a number of ways. It is not that the staff is uncaring, rather it seems that traditional ways of doing things get handed down and are seldom examined with a view to understanding their meaning or rationale. A few examples will illustrate this point. More frequently than not, holiday celebrations and decorations in nursing homes and long-term care institutions are of grade school level. Adults in a normal environment simply do not cut out Easter bunnies, red hearts, and the like and display these on their doors and windows. It is extremely difficult to maintain a sense of adult dignity in an environment in which one is addressed as deary or honey or by diminutive nicknames. Maintaining a sense of reality and holding on to the normative aspects of living becomes a most difficult task in an environment that fails to distinguish in its schedule and activities, the normal division of a day's activities such as a time and place for work, a time and place for leisure, or in the observance of a holiday on that holiday, or differentiating weekends from weekdays. Holding church services on a Friday or Monday afternoon and Jewish services on a Sunday may indeed be the most convenient arrangement for the minister or the rabbi or the church's schedule, but it certainly is not reality orienting or normalizing for the patients. Movies and bingo in the morning or early afternoon are not typical of the outside community. The message seems to be that an abnormal environment is acceptable for abnormal persons or at least, the needs and rights of staff determine schedules and program focus.

In a different context, Searles (1960) and Csikszentmihalyi and Rochberg-Halton (1981) emphasize the importance of the nonhuman environment from the perspective of individual psychology. These authors point up the significance thoughout life of an individual's relatedness to his or her nonhuman world and to the objects in that world. These transactions, they argue, between persons and things, between persons and the structure and order of their world, shape and reinforce self-identity and a sense of personal integrity. It is argued that such relatedness helps in the testing and verification of reality and in coping with threat, change, and anxieties. Such studies point up the importance of an environment that encourages having and caring for personal possessions, such as a special picture, a teacup from home, a treasured rocking chair. Lifetime possessions that represent belonging, that hold memories of family or special relationships and events are of increasing significance as one grows older. Having these close by, being able to touch them, to reminisce about them, is a crucial link with one's past and a sense of continuity in one's life. Objects that depict and verify one's competence are of particular importance to the older individual whose competencies are diminishing. Objects that the person has created, special awards and recognitions, all help to verify both to self and others one's competence, one's ability to achieve and one's connectedness with life events. An environment that provides for interactions with living things, the growing of plants, of flowers or vegetables, the caring for and relating to animals and birds, is an environment that nurtures and helps to sustain a sense of self as caringly human.

A personal identity, a sense of continuity of one's life are reinforced by the nature of one's relatedness to the structure and order of one's world. For institutionalized older adults, the fit between their characteristic lifestyle and the structure of daily living activities that characterize the institution is crucial. To achieve a positive impact, the structure and order of the institutional environment must accommodate and provide options that foster a continuity of the elderly person's lifestyle (Kiernat, 1982).

SUSTAINING FUNCTION AND INDEPENDENCE

Sensory changes occur universally in the later years of life and each individual experiences a different rate, degree, and type of loss. During the late 70's and early 80's, sensory changes begin to impact daily functioning. Tasks that were previously accomplished without thought may now require considerable concentration. Performing the activities of daily living in one's customary way may present a challenge and thus threaten the autonomy of the older person. In order to understand the ways in which the physical environment can be adapted to accommodate sensory changes and support the functioning of the older adult, it is important to understand the changes that take place in the process of aging (Colavita, 1978; Corso, 1971; Cutler, 1979; Maguire, 1985; National Council on Aging, 1985).

As age advances there are a number of ocular changes (Cristarella, 1977). The pupil of the eye decreases in size with resulting need for more light in order to distinguish objects. The density of the lens also increases and yellows, resulting in a greater scattering of light and fading of colors. The ability of the eye to focus also changes, requiring close proximity to an object before it can be identified. These changes in the eye cause the older person to have more difficulty in functioning at low light levels, adjusting to a dimly lit area after being outside or in bright light, seeing objects clearly and/or not recognizing objects until they are quite close, reading printed material, seeing cooler colors (blues and greens look faded to the older eye), experiencing glare and the scattering of light, which makes it even more difficult to see. These changes and the impact they have on the older person's functioning can cause feelings of insecurity and vulnerability in coping with the environment.

Hearing loss is one of the most frequently encountered problems of aging. There are two types of hearing impairment. One in which sound has difficulty reaching the inner ear with the result that sound intensity is lost. Hearing aides are most helpful in eliminating or reducing this problem. The other hearing loss is most characteristic of the aging process. Nerve endings in the inner ear degenerate, with resulting difficulty in perceiving and distinguishing high-frequency sounds. This impairment creates problems in comprehending speech, most especially when it is rapid and/or when words are not clearly enunciated. It is therefore difficult to follow conversations in a group when several persons are speaking simultaneously. Background noises such as television, music, or traffic mask vowel sounds and an individual with such hearing loss will not be able to fully comprehend what is being said. The hearing-impaired elder can thus experience confusion, suspiciousness, depression, and respond by withdrawal from social situations. Hearing loss can cause an older individual to begin to question his/her own mental capacity.

As one ages there is a decline in the ability to taste and smell because of progressive atrophy of taste buds and a diminution in olfactory function. The sense of taste and smell are closely related and are important in making food appealing, determining flavor, and in identifying rancid foods, leaking gas, and warnings of fire. Thus loss of these senses adversely affects the older person's appetite and warning system.

Touch is the sense that undergoes the last amount of change as one ages although there is a gradual reduction in touch sensation. Touching is a powerful means of communication, of demonstrating intimacy, caring, and friendship. It is a significant sensory stimulator and alerter. Touch is a means of orientation to space and objects, and touch and stroking play an important role in reaffirming an image of one's body. There is some reason to conjecture that touch is a stronger sense than is generally believed. The need to touch objects as a way of discovery, of exploration is quite evident in the very young, parental admonitions of "don't touch," notwithstanding. This means of gaining information diminishes as sensory, perceptual, and cognitive systems mature. However the urge for many adults to feel, to touch, for example, the smoothness of a rock, the softness of a fabric, the velvet of a petal, is clearly evident.

A decline in muscle tone and strength and disturbances in body mechanics causes problems in the orientation of one's body in space and in the ability to readily perceive changes in body position. Body balance may also prove to be a problem. These changes cause the older person to alter his or her gait and move more slowly, since a longer amount of time in contact with the ground is necessary for mobility.

In addition to sensory losses, there are some intellectual changes associated with aging (Haselkus, 1974). It is generally agreed that there is no diminution of verbal ability and that this function remains intact and is a rich resource for adaptation. In contrast, speed in intellectual processing does slow down with age. Thus it takes the older person longer to think through an issue or problem and act on it. Actual intellectual functioning is not impaired, it is the speed of problem solving that is effected. Difficulties in performing under time pressure can create a functional problem.

It must be remembered that there are vast individual differences in intellectual capacities and functioning. Changes related to aging likewise show a diverse pattern. Most of the older person's difficulty with memory seems to occur in what has been called secondary memory. This involves retention of many items that have been learned quite recently. Problems with the recall of recent events increases with pressure of time, anxiety about doing well, preoccupation and/or inattention. Problems with secondary memory can effect health and safety. For example, medication may not be taken, or taken too frequently; or the individual may fail to remember to attend to necessary precautions at the appropriate time, such as unplugging the iron, turning off the stove, and the like.

It is generally acknowledged that long-term memory holds up fairly well with age and is a significant asset in coping and adaptation, as is the capacity to learn, which continues throughout life. When the environment is responsive to such needs, it plays a significant role in helping the person learn to more effectively use his/her capacities productively to compensate for loss. However, environments with inadequate stimuli and accommodation can seriously reduce the ability to function.

Studies in sensory deprivation, (Solomen, 1961; Zabek, 1969) have demonstrated that meaningless, low-stimulus environments do cause significant behavioral deficits. In summarizing research, Parent (1978) describes four conditions that characterize such environments and the maladaptive behaviors they elicit. These include: (1) *sensory deprivation* where there is a lack of visual, auditory, tactile, and kinesthetic stimuli. These are environments characterized by poor lighting, too much or too little sound, and limited opportunity for movement. There is little to see, hear, touch, or do. In such settings there is a loss of fine-motor skills, poor concentration, disorientation in time, and loss of motivation. (2) *Perceptual deprivation* characterizes an environment that is meaningless in the sense that there are few discernible cues and a vague, drab sameness. Routines are monotonous and unvarying. There is a lack of distinction between time of day, one day from the next, or even day and night. These environments adversely affect cognitive, intellectual functioning. There is a diminution in reasoning, in space orientation and in verbal fluency. (3) *Immobilization* is characterized by severe restriction of kinesthetic stimuli. In these environments movement is very limited or restricted by the continued use of wheelchairs, Geri-chairs, bed rest, arm and/or leg casts, heavy medication, and/or a variety of body restraints. Confinement by immobilization results in impaired performance on both simple and complex tasks, a decreased dexterity and difficulty in thinking. (4) *Social isolation* can result from hearing loss, speech disorders, and language barriers that make communication difficult. In addition, the confinement of patients to private rooms; the placement of furniture in linear, classroom, or airport fashion, rather than in circles or face-to-face; noise that precludes speaking and hearing; or large open spaces are environmental elements that encourage withdrawal and isolate behaviors. In these environments there is an increasing sense of loneliness, hostility, temporal disorientation, rumination, and discouragement.

ENVIRONMENTAL ADAPTATION

It becomes clear that the environment is a critical dynamic in shaping behavior (Weinberg, 1970; Crowhurst, 1975; Attal, 1987) In work with the elderly, it is especially important that the environment be planned and shaped to maximize functioning. Lindsley (1964) has used the term "prosthetic environments" to describe those settings where accommodations are made to compensate for changes that occur with aging. Some of the important adaptations that should be considered include the following.

Lighting

Appropriate lighting is essential in helping to compensate for the changes that occur in vision and hearing. Each room requires multiple sources of sufficiently bright light. Varied light sources help create an even level of illumination without extremely bright or dark spots. To reduce glare and the scattering of light, sheer shades or curtains that can be used with draperies allow light to enter a room but act as a filter to reduce glare. The strategic placement of table and floor lamps help to provide an even level of light and creates a warm, home-like atmosphere. Adequate lighting without shadows is also important for the hearing impaired, as being able to see facial features and expression aids in communication.

The entrance to buildings should be well lit with natural and/or artificial illumination to reduce the hazards of the blinding that can occur when one comes in from the glare of bright sunlight to a shaded area. The glare from highly glossed and polished tile floors can be treacherous for the older person, particularly when there is a source of light reflecting on the floor (Wilmont, 1986). Carpeting eliminates this problem but may create its own problems in terms of maintenance. In areas where discolorations and soiling are most likely to happen, a tile floor may be the wisest choice. Some tile materials and colors have less gloss than others. A new type of carpeting is beginning to appear on the market. These products are made of 12″ × 12″ squares easily removed for spot cleaning and then replaced. Although the initial cost is high, these carpets are attractive and significantly reduce the problem of maintenance. Another concern related to lighting is the number of falls that occur in bedrooms and baths as the older person navigates between the two at night. Night lights and bedside flashlights significantly reduce such risks.

Color

Color plays an important role both in assisting the older person to manage his/her environment and in creating an attractive setting. It is important to keep in mind that the cooler colors such as pale blues and greens tend to fade away to the older eye and are thus difficult to distinguish. More intense shades of blue and green and the warmer reds, oranges, yellows, pinks, and browns are better choices. It is preferable for wall colors to contrast with the floor coloring because such contrast helps to distinguish the boundaries of a room. Likewise, doorways should contrast with walls. Different-colored doorways help disoriented patients identifying their rooms. The use of contrasting colors on food trays, so that dishes can by readily distinguished from the tray surface, helps the patient to manage independent eating and adds an important element of attractiveness to the food being served.

The tunnel effect and disorientating quality of long corridors can be mitigated by the use of different color tones on the walls to break up the space and reduce the sense of vastness. Color is furthermore useful as a means of orienting patients to their surroundings and providing directions to given areas. Attractive graphics, painted in contrasting colors on hallway walls can point the way to the dining room, living units, the auditorium, coffee shop, and the like. Each patient living unit decorated in a different color scheme and related decor, such as colonial, provincial, traditional, will identify each unit and its uniqueness. In order to feel secure in moving about and leaving an area, the patient must be sure of his/her ability to return to his space.

Lettering

One of the most common complaints among older persons is the inability to distinguish letters and therefore read written material. The lettering on rooms, signs, elevators, mailboxes, menus, newsletters, notices, and so forth must be sufficiently large and well spaced in order for the older person to be able to comfortably read. The enlargement of printed material should include an increase in the height and width of the lettering as well as greater spacing between letters. The paper used for written material should be in a warm tone such as beige, off-white, yellow, and on matte paper. Letters and numbers should appear in sharp contrast to their background; this is particularly important in marking appliances with on/off or hot/cold switches as well as for all fire and safety precautions. The environment should, of course, offer a wide variety of large-print books and magazines.

Sound

The inability to hear clearly is another common complaint among older persons. There are a number of actions that can be taken to assist the older person in communication. Lighting, as we have mentioned, is an important factor as it enables the older person to see facial expressions and to watch lip movements, thus providing additional cues as to what is being said. When speaking with a person who is hearing impaired, it is helpful to face the person directly, speak at a slower pace and use distinct pronunciation. In addition, signaling changes in the conversation and encouraging repetition if something is not understood, will result in a better understanding of what is being said. Background noise can be a significant contributor to the disorientation of the patient. For example, on one patient living unit, there was a bedside radio in each room, placed there for the patient's pleasure and for sensory stimulation. Staff attending to the patient would turn on the radios when they entered the rooms. What resulted was a variety of rock music coming from different rooms at high volume. Communication between patient and staff was difficult at best and the music was neither age or culturally relevant. Music became an irritating noise. The young staff simply needed to be reminded of the hearing problems of the elderly and the difficulties they have with sensory overload in order for the problem to be corrected. Intercoms and over-used public address systems, as well as piped in music, are other examples of distracting and frequently confusing background noise.

The telephone can be another frustrating experience for the hearing impaired. It may be difficult to hear the caller and there are no visual cues to assist in deciphering the message.

Telephones in hallways or areas of movement and activity present a particular problem. Amplifiers on these instruments are critical to their use. In addition, large-print overlays on dials help to identify letters and numbers and thus encourage the use of the instruments. Whenever possible telephones should be located in areas that are quiet and that provide some privacy.

Touch

Because touch remains relatively intact, it can and should be used to compensate for other sensory loss. Texture can be used to help to identify and navigate the environment, such as textured elevator buttons, wall light switches, and the like. Touchable wall hangings and pictures that include a variety of fabrics, pebbles, metal and similar materials, and smooth and textured fabrics on furnishings are all ways of being responsive to many elderly individuals' strong need for touch. Games and activities that involve identifying a wide variety of objects by touch without benefit of sight are a great source of pleasure in touching and sharing with others. Massage is a striking use of touch in sustaining and enhancing one's body image. It is truly unfortunate that massage and back rubs are not regularly provided. Likewise, opportunities to hold and stroke animals, to have and/or collect objects that can be touched and retouched are ways of being responsive to this need. To touch and to be touched is an important means of obtaining information about one's environment and about one's self.

Safety Issues

There are a number of issues to be considered in creating an environment to ensure security and safety. The decrease in sensitivity to tilt that occurs with aging increases the possibility of falling. This factor, in combination with the diminution of muscle strength, makes the availability of handrails and grab bars essential. Handrails are necessary in any area where there is required ambulation for any distance and in areas where maintaining balance may be difficult, such as stairs, ramps, bathrooms, and showers. Door handles with a latch movement rather than a turning knob facilitate movement through doorways. Well-illuminated crosswalks and outdoor stairs are a necessity as steps can be a hazard unless they are clearly marked. Painting the first and last step of a stairway in bright colors can aid in depth perception. The edges of individual steps marked with a bright contrasting color aids in negotiating stairs because such markings help in discerning where a step ends. The clear marking of appliances in the kitchen and in bathrooms is critical in order for the individual to be able to readily distinguish between on and off, hot or cold.

The problem of retaining the confused wandering patient in a safe environment without serious limits to mobility or the restriction of others can be handled by the use of an electronic sensor. There are many such systems available. They allow as much freedom to the individual as possible and eliminate the use of restrictive measures, such as locked doors, confinement to a room, Geri-chairs, or chemical restraints.

SOME PSYCHO-SOCIAL COMPONENTS OF THE ENVIRONMENT

The use of space is an expression of beliefs, expectations, and function. The architectural structure, furnishings, light, color, temperature, odor, sound, and order all shape the atmosphere (Wolfensberger, 1972; Kramer & Kramer, 1976; Kiernat, 1982). As pointed out earlier, the total atmosphere has an impact on the way staff, patients, and visitors interact, react, and perceive themselves within the context of the environment and the mission of the facility.

The structure and use of space can create social and psychologic barriers or it can encourage and foster social interaction and emphasize living and doing. Designs and arrangements can encourage persons to keep apart from one another and emphasize the value of privacy and separateness. Long, unbroken corridors, seating arrangements in rows such as a waiting room or terminal, closed doors and partitions all relay the same message. On the other hand, furniture arranged in clusters or circles, open doors, and the elimination of partitions encourages socialization. When the glass partitions that surrounded the nursing stations in one of the buildings in our facility were removed, there was a significant change in the feeling, tone, and level of interaction between patient and staff on those units.

The location of certain areas of patient activity as well as their design is an important factor. There are natural gathering areas in all facilities and the challenge is to maximize their socialization potential. Experience demonstrates that basement or penthouse areas or rooms isolated by long corridors, no matter how attractive, will be underutilized. They are simply too far removed from the mainstream of activity for either patients or staff. Lobbies and entrance ways where people who are coming and going can be seen and greeted are natural congregating areas. Again, as an example, in our facility, patients regularly congregated just inside the entrance way, which was also adjacent to the nurses' station. Although a day room had been designed at the back end of each of the units, no amount of cajoling or pressure could dissuade the patients from moving their chairs and gathering in the entrance way. These areas would become congested and constitute a fire hazard. The purchase of furniture typical of a family room and its clustering to accommodate to traffic, safety concerns, and the social interest of patients resolved the issue.

There are some additional considerations when areas are being created to promote socialization. The arrangement of furniture must allow for the free movement of wheelchairs. For the elderly population, it is especially important that furniture be arranged so that individuals can see clearly those individuals with whom they are speaking. Hearing impairments make this essential. Carpeting helps to make social areas more invitingly warm and absorbs sound. If incontinence is an issue then the newer, more easily maintained carpet squares or vinyl tiles are of course a wiser choice.

The use of Naugahyde or a similar covering for chairs and

sofas in many institutions seems to be the traditional way of coping with problems of incontinence, food spills, and cigarette burns. One strong objection to this solution is that it removes responsibility from the patient for his/her behavior. At the same time it makes a statement of staff's expectations regarding patient behaviors. In addition, the material is cold and lacking in texture. We believe both of these are counterproductive. Continence management programs, the use of Attends® or similar products as well as programs aimed at increasing and supporting the patient's sense of adult responsibility do indeed work positively for both patients and staff. Additionally, cloth fabrics (as we have pointed out) are important in sensory processing and provide a wide variety of decorative color and design with a sense of warmth and attractiveness. To make the use of fabrics practical, a piece of plastic can be inserted between the cushions of chairs and sofas and their outer covering. Decorative fabrics can then be used over the plastic as a cover, sprayed with Scotch Guard®, and removed for cleaning.

For the elderly, furniture must be chosen with a view toward the ease of getting in and out of a sitting position. Thus the availability of two sturdy arm rests is essential and chairs and loveseats are preferable to sofas. We have found that when chair seats are raised to 17½ inches and coffee tables to 21 inches, the older person is better able to manage. One further point, when ordering furniture, extra parts such as table tops and spindles can frequently be purchased. This allows for inexpensive and immediate repairs rather than replacement when parts are broken or become obsolete.

The appeal of eating and sharing food with others is universal. It is a traditional means of engaging and sharing with others. Food is to be enjoyed in the company of others. The diminution of appetite, the loss of interest in food that seems to regularly accompany solitary meals is evidence of the strong social and interpersonal components of eating. As an individual ages, mealtimes are replete with symbolic meaning, with memories of celebrations, of special events, and shared times with family and friends. Specific foods are frequently associated with memorable events in both a positive or negative sense. For the institutionalized elderly, dining is particularly important and should be one of the most significant daily living activities of the institution. Its potential as a therapeutic, health-sustaining agent cannot be overemphasized. The food itself, its taste and appearance, how and when it is offered and the setting in which meals occur are the elements that determine the critical nature of dining.

It was not surprising therefore that meal service and the environment of the dining room were one of the first areas for scrutiny and change. The institution's dining room had been essentially unchanged for approximately 50 years. It was a cavernous, institutional space, noisy, cold, and most unattractive. Painting the walls a warm color with a darker shade at each end of the room, arranging tables and chairs in clusters rather than in the traditional institutional linear pattern, reduced the cavernous quality and projected a sense of warmth. Old furniture was replaced with small round or square oak tables with formica centers matching the warm wall color, and oak chairs with arms for ease in sitting and rising. Patient's art work was framed and hung and many plants from the newly developing patient-run greenhouse were added to complete the decor. The transformation was marked as was the response of patients and staff.

Changing food-service patterns and schedules in order to promote a more normalizing environment and experience proved, of course, to be more of a challenge than improving the physical environment of the dining room. The first change was to establish the expectation that all patients would eat in the dining room unless of course they were too ill to leave their rooms or beds. It had become common practice for those patients residing in the skilled nursing building to take their meals on their floor or in their rooms. This practice, we believed, was a contributing factor to staff and patients' feelings of isolation, to the sense of patient invalidism, and dependency. There were limited opportunities for contact outside the parameters of the building and in many respects the building had become a total institution. Having staff and patients use the main dining room helped to break the isolation, extending opportunities for socialization and healthier patterns of functioning. For those who were temporarily unable to manage the dining room, a congregate eating area on the unit was established. With very few exceptions, patients did not eat alone. Such change required alterations in habitual patterns and schedules as well as in attitudes about patient capacities and interests. Initially, many nursing staff viewed these breaks with tradition as uncaring, as reflecting a disregard for patient comfort and safety. It was many, many months before such change became the accepted pattern and was acknowledged as positive.

A second factor that required attention was the flexibility of dining room schedules. The time allotted for meals was so condensed that long lines would form waiting to reach the serving area. Eating had become a rushed affair rather than a leisurely pleasure. Dining hours for each unit were expanded and patients who did not require escort service were extended the privilege of eating at any time during dining room hours. This was a new privilege valued and coveted by patients but again viewed warily by some of the staff who doubted the patients' ability to be independently responsible. These doubts were short lived, however, and the success of this initiative paved the way for the creation of a small patient smoking section in the dining room. Patients who demonstrated responsibility were given the privilege of sitting in this special section and having a cigarette after a meal, unattended by staff, and using their own lighter or matches. This privilege meant a great deal to the patient, it reinforced adult responsibility and was not abused.

Other changes that focused on increasing patient autonomy and the normalization of the environment included the choice of sleeping in on a weekend and having a continental breakfast on the floor or of going to the dining room for a full breakfast. Special efforts were made to clearly distinguish holiday meals from those regularly served. The food-service staff came to take great pride in providing for special occasions such as family meals on Thanksgiving and Christmas. On these days and other special occasions, color-coordinated cloth napkins and table covers with relevant centerpieces became a standard practice. Patients organized a committee to create the centerpieces for each holiday and to work with food-service staff in preparing decorative dining room decor. For those patients whose eating behaviors were disturbing to others, or a danger to themselves, a group was established called Delicate Dining. This group sat at a special table in the dining room where they were coached by staff, encouraged and rewarded for demonstrating safe, socially acceptable eating habits. For individuals who had spent most of their adult lives in state institutions and whose eating habits were essentially ignored, such achievement was noteworthy.

The celebration of holidays in an institution is as we have pointed out earlier, a special concern. The opportunity for patients to celebrate those holidays that are important to them in the culturally relevant ways that have been part of their lifestyle, is critical to the quality of their life in the institution, to their sense of satisfaction, and to their state of health. The celebration of a holiday, like the differentiation of days and weekends, is a critical reality-orienting experience, acknowledging and marking the flow of seasons, the distinction of days, and eliciting learned behavioral patterns associated with the healthy aspects of self. Additionally, activities that mark a special day or seasonal change, and which are culture and age relevant reinforce the sense of personal identity.

Characteristically, holidays in institutions are times when there is minimal staff coverage and such coverage is usually understood to be the sole responsibility of nursing. Thus there is generally a skeleton staff, devoid of professionals except for nurses at times when the patient is most apt to feel a sense of loss and need support and help in coping. Furthermore, in many systems, it is common practice to accommodate holiday time off for staff by celebrating a holiday on a regular weekday rather than on the holiday. Programming for patients thus comes to be based on management or staff interests rather than on the needs and interests of patients. To compound the problems of holidays, it is generally accepted that the clinical professional staff do not become involved in holiday activities. When such activities occur on a regular workday, it is common practice for this staff to maintain their regular workday schedules and role functions. We firmly believe that these practices are not responsive to the needs of patients, are time disorienting and certainly do not reflect or support the sense of community and shared responsibility for the total operations of an institution.

In our setting, it was clear that change was needed and new policies were subsequently developed. These included the expectation that all holidays would be celebrated on the actual holiday, that all clinical staff would share responsibility for holiday activities, and that the activities planned would reflect patient interests, culture, and adulthood. To implement this policy, a holiday-planning committee was established with representatives from each patient unit and each clinical discipline. The responsibility of the committee was to prepare a total plan for each holiday throughout the year including staff schedules and participation, the nature of the total day and its special activities. A rotation schedule was collaboratively developed for clinical staff and each staff became involved in planning and participating in the events of the day for which they, their colleagues, and the patients carried responsibility. The change in feeling and the quality of holiday celebrations was of course, marked. Nursing staff commented again and again about how their feelings of isolation and "being dumped on" had been replaced by a sense of sharing and a concern from and about others. Feedback from patients and staff emphasized the different and broadened perspectives they gained by seeing one another in different settings and circumstances. The concept of the total person in his/her total environment had begun to move beyond words toward the reality of action.

SUSTAINING CHANGE

Maintaining the esthetic and therapeutic qualities of the environment is an ongoing process. It requires regular monitoring, collaborative, and coordinated efforts among maintenance, housekeeping, and clinical staff. The traditional "tugs of war" between maintenance and clinical staff are, of course, counterproductive. Our efforts to address these concerns resulted in the creation of a top management position of Environmental Coordinator. This position carried responsibility for the overall coordination of the planning and maintenance of all aspects of the physical environment to ensure that it maximized patient and staff functioning and was esthetically pleasing. To ensure full collaboration, an environmental committee was formed with representation from the maintenance and housekeeping departments, the patient council, clinical, and other staff. Some of the principle initiatives that were undertaken included: the setting of priorities and the development and implementation of a refurbishing and redecorating plan for all patient and staff areas throughout the institution; development of schedules for the monitoring and routine repainting, repair, and maintenance of areas; responsibility for the purchase of all furnishings and an inventory of all furnishings; the review and assessment of the use of all space and development of a plan for the allocation of space to enhance function; and plans for monitoring safety, lighting, temperature, sound, cleanliness and the use of space, particularly in patient areas. In essence, the coordinator and the committee were empowered to put into place a system that would generate a responsive, attractive, and accommodating environment and ensure insofar as possible, the endurance of such qualities.

The nonhuman or physical environment has many facets and meanings. It has a marked impact on the purpose of an institution, on the performance of patients and staff and on the quality of life within the institution. In this chapter we have attempted to explain and demonstrate ways in which the environment (a) reflects attitudes, beliefs, values, and expectations regarding the provider and the consumer of the services that are provided; (b) can through the real and symbolic meaning of things and rituals, provide opportunity for verifying and reaffirming personal identity, value and a continuity of life; and (c) can through its structure and order, sustain function, enable a sense of independence and competence and sustain health.

Throughout this chapter we have emphasized that a state of health, a sense of well-being is defined by the nature of the relationship between an individual's capacities and the nature of that person's external world. With the advancement of age or the existence of an illness, capacities tend to diminish. When the environment is designed to be responsive to individual needs, capacities and limitations, when it clarifies reality, the capacity to cope and the sense of personal identity is supported and the quality of life is enhanced.

REFERENCES

Attal, D. (1987). The senior dilemma: Alternative services for older adults. *The Forum, 11*(28), 3–5.

Colavita, F. B. (1978). *Sensory changes in the elderly.* Springfield, IL: Charles C Thomas.

Corso, J. (1971). Sensory processes of age effects in normal adults. *Journal of Gerontology, 26*(1), 90–105.

Cristarella, M. C. (1977). Visual functions of the elderly. *American Journal of Occupational Therapy, 37*(7), 432–445.

Crowhurst, S. D. (1975). Reawakening senses in the elderly. *Canadian Nursing, 71,* 22.

Csikszentmihalyi, M., & Rochberg-Halton, E. (1981). *The meaning of things domestic symbols and the self.* New York: Cambridge University Press.

Cutler, S. C. (1979). *The mature years.* New Jersey: Charles B. Slack.

Goffman, I. (1961). *Asylums.* New York: Anchor Books. Doubleday.

Haselkus, B. R. (1974). Aging and the human nervous system. *American Journal Occupational Therapy, 28*(1), 16–21.

Kiernat, J. (1982). Environment: The hidden modality. *Physical and Occupational Therapy in Geriatrics, 2*(1), 3–12.
Kiernat, J. M. (1985). Environmental aspects affecting health. In Maguire, G. H., (Ed.), *Care of the elderly*. Boston: Little Brown.
Kramer, C. H., & Kramer, J. R. (1976). *Developing a therapeutic community*. Springfield, IL: Charles C Thomas.
Langer, E. I., & Rodin, J. (1976). The effects of choice and enhanced personal responsibility for the aged. A field experiment in an institutional setting. *Journal of Personality and Social Psychology, 34,* 191–198.
Lindsley, O. R. (1964). Geriatric behavior prosthetics. In R. Kastenbaum (Ed.), *New thoughts on old age*. New York: Springer Publishing Co.
Maier, S. F., & Seligman, M.E.P. (1976). Learned helplessness: Theory and evidence. *Journal of Experimental Psychology, 105,* 3–46.
Maguire, G. H. (Ed.). (1985). *Care of the elderly: A health team approach*. Boston, Little Brown.
National Council on Aging, Inc. (1985). *The Sixth Sense. Understanding sensory changes and aging*. Washington, DC:
Parent, L. H. (1978). Effects of a low-stimulus environment on behavior. *American Journal of Occupational Therpay, 32*(1), 19–25.
Searles, H. (1960). *The non-human environment*. New York: International Universities Press.
Sherman, E., & Newman, E. S. (1977). The meaning of cherished personal possessions for the elderly. *Journal of Aging and Human Development, 8*(2), 181–192.
Solomen, P. (1961). *Sensory deprivation*. Cambridge, MA: Harvard University Press.
Weinberg, J. (1970). Environment, Its language and the aging. *Journal of American Geriatric Society, 18,* 681.
Wilmont, M. (1986). The effect of a vinyl floor surface and carpeted floor surface upon walking in elderly hospital in-patients. *Age and Aging, 15,* 119–120.
Wolfensberger, W. (1972). *Normalization*. National Institute on Mental Retardation. York University, Toronto, Canada.
Zabek, J. P. (1969). *Sensory deprivation: Fifteen years of research*. New York: Appleton Century Crofts.

Interdisciplinary Functional Skills-Assessment Methodology

5

RATIONALE

For at least the past two decades, significant changes have occurred in how mental illness is understood and defined and therefore which interventions are viewed as having credibility and assigned priority by society, by professionals, and by delivery systems. The definition and treatment of mental illness are not static phenomena. Throughout history, as well as now, such constructs have been shaped by the social, cultural, and economic factors of the time in relation to existing knowledge and technology.

Deinstitutionalization was part of this evolutionary process and the fundamental reconstruction of ideology in the mental health system. The advent of chemotherapy and the consciousness raising of the 1960s with its emphasis on patient rights and treatment in the least restrictive setting ushered in the era of deinstitutionalization. The resulting dramatic increase in the number of psychiatrically disabled persons in the community brought into sharp focus the serious dysfunctions of this population.

Data from the mid-1980s (Brady, 1984; Cohen & Anthony, 1984; Goldman, Gattozzi, & Taube, 1981; Kuehnel, DeRisi, &

Lieberman, 1983) indicate that 50% to 60% of discharged patients cannot sustain life in the community for two years. Only 10% are employed and 71% rarely or never engage in recreation with others (Cohen & Anthony, 1984). In a sample of patients with both high and low recidivism rates, both groups were rated as needing assistance in bathing, dressing, and grooming. Less than 10% of both groups were judged able to maintain a home or apartment, keep appointments, or hold a paying job (Goldman, Gattozzi, & Taube, 1981). When the process of aging is added to the chronic illness, the problems of functioning are compounded.

The prevalence and severity of deficits in community living skills continues to challenge our traditional methods and perspectives of treatment priorities and needs. Reality has brought sharply into focus the inadequacy of only treating the illness and controlling symptoms while neglecting to address the urgent need for functional skill development.

Gittleman and Friedman (1988) confront mental health professionals with treating only half of the illness and neglecting to attend to the rehabilitation needs of patients. This omission, these authors point out, has resulted in a population of mentally ill who are considerably disabled and unable to care for themselves. Brief hospitalization usually leaves patients with residual symptoms and serious functional deficits. Treatment and rehabilitation programs within the hospital targeted to preparing patients for postinstitutional environments are essential (Kuehnel et al., 1983)

Brooks (1981) has graphically depicted the responsibility of the hospital in preparing patients to cope with life in the community. He has stated "the first order of business in deinstitutionalization is getting the institution out of the person. Only secondarily should we be concerned with getting the person out of the institution. Simply controlling symptoms and placing individuals in less restrictive environments is a gross disservice. . . ." Minkoff (1987) suggests that an extended initial period of hospitalization can facilitate a more stable adaptation to illness. Research has demonstrated that the degree to which deinstitutionalization is successful, depends in good measure on systematic assessment, treatment, and rehabilitation procedures within the hospital, targeted to preparing patients for postinstitutional environments. (Kuehnel et al., 1983; Paul & Lentz, 1977; Brady, 1984).

For the mentally ill elderly the importance of a functional skill assessment must be accentuated. For the long-term mentally ill who have grown old in the system, the limitations imposed by adjustment to institutional life, the residuals of a psychosis, and the aging process are evident. Functional skills learning is essential if life outside an institution is to be realized. For those who will remain in the protective environment of an institution, the comprehensive functional skill-assessment methodology does indeed increase the chances that services and programs will be individually relevant and that the quality of life will be enhanced.

The mandate for comprehensive, systematic assessment and systematic interventions based on assessments places a critical significance on interdisciplinary collaboration. It requires a truly interactive process of problem solving and consensus building, a respect for one anothers discipline-specific knowledge and expertise and a shared concept of the meaning and ultimate importance of the total patient and the total environment. Implicit is a commitment to a shared responsibility for ensuring that the total needs of the patient are addressed in an integrated manner and that the total environment is responsive and relevant to such needs.

A Comprehensive Functional Skills Assessment model is an interdisciplinary process and method for identifying, categorizing, and measuring those performance skills and functions deemed necessary for community living. It is an organizing structure for pooling and interrelating discipline-specific information and perspectives, for reaching consensus, planning interventions, and evaluating outcomes. It provides measurable indicators for both treatment and rehabilitation initiatives and enables the design of explicitly relevant programs with measurable goals.

The use of a measured assessment reduces the subjectivity of some of the assumptions we tend to make regarding program needs of patients. For example, in one setting there was agreement among members of the treatment team that the priority need of the community living skills program they were planning was the development of work skills, attitudes, and habits. Such an assumption seemed reasonable because the targeted population was comprised of working-age males with a history of long-term hospitalization. Data from the functional skills assessment, however, challenged this assumption, indicating that the top priority for this group was managing stress. Similarly, assumptions about the cognitive functional limitations of a group of chronically mentally ill elderly were not substantiated by the functional skills assessment data.

In a different context, the economic, social, and political pressures to verify the efficacy of treatment adds to the value and usefulness of the comprehensive functional skills assessment. Quality assurance is one of the highest priorities in the health care system today. The critical focus on documenting the relevance of intervention in relation to definable needs and goals are only two examples of the requirements for accountability. The functional skills assessment is without question, a valuable and viable method and process for meeting such quality assurance requirements.

COMPONENTS OF A COMPREHENSIVE ASSESSMENT

Functional skills assessments have traditionally been seen as a rehabilitation process, frequently separate from the focus and orientation of the psychiatric diagnosis and its related treatment procedures. The extent to which efforts have been made to interrelate these two perspectives has depended on the philosophy and treatment orientation of the setting and/or the nature of the patient population. Patient characteristics (acute or chronic) are frequently the determining factor in the choice of one focus over the other, in contrast to combining or interrelating the two orientations. However, new approaches to problem solving as well as changes in the nature of the problems confronting the system today, are changing our perspectives. General systems theory has altered our way of thinking and our understanding of the interrelationships of events. Deinstitutionalization has made visible the dramatic numbers and serious problems of psychiatrically disabled persons. As a result, both professionals and society have begun to redefine the issues and the optimum system required to improve them. Change is more and more evident in current literature. There are increasing references to psychiatric rehabilitation, psychosocial rehabilitation, and functional skills assessment. Furthermore, the fact that traditional diagnoses are becoming more behaviorally descriptive reflects the current emphasis on function.

A comprehensive interdisciplinary assessment methodology brings together psychiatric and rehabilitation orientations to ensure that the needs and goals of the patient are systematically and relevantly addressed in an integrated manner. The end goal of such an endeavor is to help the patient sustain a life style outside of an institution that is more satisfying than not to self and significant others. To support this goal an assessment must be comprehensive. It must address all behaviors that significantly impact the ability to function in the community (Anthony, Cohen, & Cohen, 1984; Cohen & Anthony, 1984; Fidler, 1984).

Manifest behaviors are the result of an individual's neurobiology, the expectations and requirements of the environment, the individual's self-esteem system and his or her repertoire of coping skills. These are dynamic, interactive elements. The sense of self and the acquisition of coping skills emerge from the nature and kind of encounter with ones external environment. The quality of such encounters, the resulting success or failure, is in relation to the nature of the demands or expectations of the environment and the characteristics and qualities of the individual's neurobiologic system, its capacities and limitations for response. Thus, successful community living depends on the functional capacities and needs of the individual in relation to the responsive capacities of the community. The pattern of failure in the lives of those who are chronically mentally ill understandably results in poor self-esteem, a sense of incompetence, a paucity of coping skills with the attendant hopelessness, depression, lack of motivation, denial, and avoidance. The psychiatric diagnosis, however, is not predictive of outcomes. There are, for example, many persons with schizophrenia who do cope in the outside world. There are many others who repeatedly fail. A person is indeed more than his illness (Fine, 1980). The science and art of the remediation process is the matching of capacity with expectation. This congruence enables successful relearning, interrupting the cycle of failure and maladaptation.

The construct and use of a comprehensive functional skills assessment must be based on a systems perspective of human performance. The challenge for us is to identify and behaviorally define those components that should be considered as the precursors or antecedents of functional skills as well as those community living skills that are deemed essential to an adaptive life outside of an institution. Addressing the components and precursors of performance is furthermore crucial to understanding which deficits can probably be remedied and which ones in all probability will need to be compensated for an accommodated.

A comprehensive functional skills assessment instrument should therefore make it possible to: (1) identify, measure, and assess the nature and level of those intact strengths and capacities, deficits and disabilities that impact performance of community daily living skills and (2) indicate the focus and priorities of interventions, remediation, and learning (Fidler, 1982; Fidler & Fidler, 1978). The instrument will thus address and measure function in two major categories of performance:

1. The components or precursors of performance, including at least the following domains:
   a. sensory-motor integration and perception;
   b. physical capacity such as health, endurance, mobility, vision, hearing;
   c. cognitive functioning;
   d. affective characteristics such as response to stress, self-esteem, assertiveness, motivation, attitudes, and feelings.

2. Community living skills relative to:
   a. self-care and self-maintenance;
   b. work and work-related capacities;
   c. leisure interests and patterns;
   d. social, interpersonal functioning.

PRINCIPLES OF A FUNCTIONAL SKILLS ASSESSMENT

Cohen and Anthony (1984) Fidler (1978) and Fidler and Fidler (1984) have articulated a number of principles that define the focus and parameters of a functional skills assessment. We have borrowed heavily from these, expanded on some, and added others as we developed our model.

1. A comprehensive assessment must be congruent with the institution's treatment and rehabilitation frame of reference. It is the overall treatment frame of reference that provides the orientation from which a comprehensive assessment is developed and implemented. When the content focus of the assessment matches the institution's ideology, a sense of collective ownership and collaborative commitment on the part of staff and patients are most likely. On the other hand, when functional skills assessment is limited to one discipline or to one aspect of patient functioning, comprehensiveness is lost. There is, furthermore, a risk of fragmented endeavors, of confusing or conflicting messages to patients and to staff regarding outcome expectations, priorities, and values.

2. A functional skills assessment should be comprehensive. If the goal of treatment and rehabilitation is to enable the patient to cope with and manage the everyday tasks and activities of living, then a functional skills assessment must address all aspects of performance. These will include those physical, cognitive, psychological, social, and interpersonal functions that impact performance as well as an assessment of community living skills.

In addition, to be comprehensive, an assessment requires the special knowledge and perspective that characterize each discipline. A total view of the patient emerges as the unique perspectives of the rehabilitation disciplines, psychiatry, nursing, social work, psychology, and the patient are pooled and interrelated. The sum is indeed greater than its parts.

3. Functional skills assessment will identify strengths, abilities, and capacities. The assessment should provide measures of intact abilities so that individualized goals as well as broader program design can reinforce and use strengths as bridges to new adaptations, enhance self-regard, and sense of personal satisfaction. Treatment environments all too frequently focus almost exclusively on deficits and dysfunction. Experience indicates that the identification and explicit use of the patient's strengths does not seem to come easily to treatment teams.

4. Skills must be defined in behavioral terms. In order for a skill to be assessed, it must be observable. A feeling state, an attitude, a motivation, for example can be assessed only as it is manifested behaviorally. A skill must be expressed in the language of action.

5. A numerical measure greatly facilitates the preparation of a population profile, the identification of indicators for program focus and priorities as well as for program evaluation. The quantitative measure of skills is very useful in documenting patient progress and providing the patient with concrete evidence of achievement.

6. The functional skills assessment should provide indicators for the design and evaluation of programs. The collective data from individual assessments gives a profile of the patient population. The data should identify the particular needs of the population, the level of such needs, and thus the resources that will be needed to programmatically address such needs. Periodic collection and analysis of individual assessment data will reflect changes in the population and indicate a need for reassessment and change in program design.

7. Functional skills assessment must always be individualized. The assessment must measure the functional abilities and deficits of each individual patient. This data should identify specific needs, the unique nature and level of such needs and provide indicators for establishing goals and priority of interventions for a given patient. Such assessment establishes criteria for assessing individual progress and for evaluating the effectiveness of interventions.

Individualized goals, however, will have realistic meaning only to the degree that they relate to both the expectations and the supportive potential of the environment in which the patient will live. What are the resources of the family or family substitute? What can the family give or manage? What does the family require of a member? What does the community offer and expect? And what are the resources, the functional capacities of the patient? These are the questions that should govern treatment and rehabilitation decisions for each patient. Individualizing treatment goals therefore require a community resource assessment. This assessment should include at least: (a) an analysis of the characteristics of the family or family surrogate, its composition, life-style patterns, social and cultural norms, patterns of caring and support, family member role expectations and responsibilities, and financial resources, (b) evaluation of the community, its social, cultural and economic standards, available social and welfare services, affiliation and leisure resources and opportunities and the accessibility of each of these. See figure 5.1, p. 77.

Individualized goals for the patient result from comparative evaluation of the interrelationships of the community, the family, and the patient's functional capacities. Successful community living depends on the congruence among these. The patients functional abilities and limitations will determine the environmental resources that will be needed. Assessment of the environment will point up those skills that will be required of the patient for successful coping. The importance of individualizing goals and programs from this point of reference cannot be overemphasized. The differing life styles for example of an independent living environment, foster care, boarding home, or a shared apartment require different functional skills. Failure to accommodate to this reality in programs and goal setting creates a risk of maladaptive responses. For example, the relevance of meal planning, food shopping, and preparation for the potential boarding home resident or the activities of daily living (ADL) kitchen equipped with dishwasher and garbage disposal for the innercity resident is counterproductive. By the same token, leisure activities customarily offered within an institution are frequently unrelated to the realities of the opportunities or life style of the patient's community environment.

8. Functional skill assessments are most useful when the patient is actively involved in the assessment and goal setting. The assessment is an especially effective tool for facilitating the patient's participation in treatment planning and in the treatment and rehabilitation processes. The patient's involvement in the plan and its implementation is essential, the tangible measures of the assessment are clarified and an incentive for participation, is enhanced more frequently than not.

9. A comprehensive assessment methodology requires the active participation and contribution of all disciplines directly involved with the patient. It is an interdisciplinary endeavor! Each discipline has its own special area of expertise and information-gathering

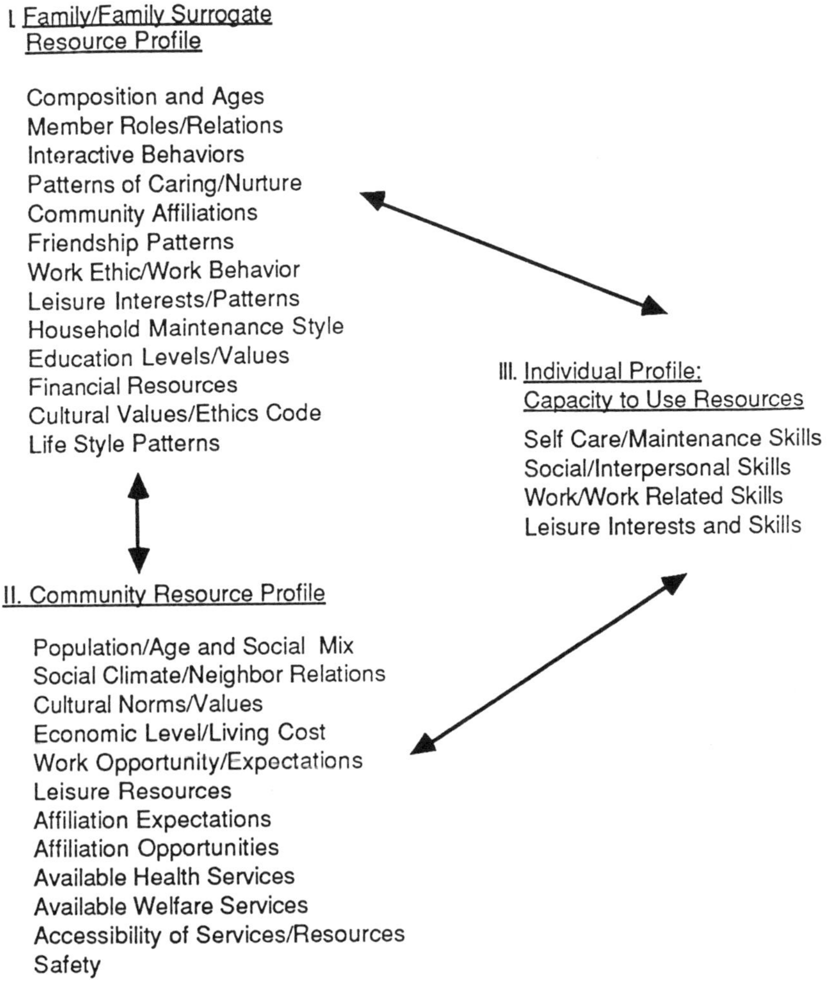

Figure 5.1 Community/individual resource assessment.

methods. Each offers a unique perspective and body of information. Discipline-specific evaluations are essential to the process of formulating a comprehensive functional skill assessment. Such assessments should reflect a consensus of the interdisciplinary staff in concert with the patient. It is a composite of interdisciplinary perspectives and judgments. The process is collaborative and interactive. The efficacy of the assessment will depend on the quality of the interaction, the quality of the discipline-specific evaluations, and the inclusion of all disciplines in the formulations. Interdisciplinary consensus regarding goal focus and outcome expectations increases the possibility of consistent reinforcement for the patient, and the creation of a responsive environment for the learning and practice of skills. Collaboration is likewise essential to the design and implementation of programs and in the quality of monitoring procedures.

One further point needs to be reemphasized. The "how" of enabling skill development, learning, or acquisition will depend on the orientation and philosophy of the setting. As Cohen and Anthony (1984) emphasises the functional skills assessment establishes the "what" not the "how."

10. Interdisciplinary staff training is a critical component of the comprehensive assessment model. The continuing development of a viable, collaborative, interactive team process is essential. Training in team building, the processes of problem identification and resolution, communication, reaching consensus and other aspects of collaborative endeavor is a critical component. It is important to remember that the success of the comprehensive assessment model or any major endeavor is in relationship to the commitment of those with top decision-making authority. It is, therefore, crucial that the overall planning, implementation, and monitoring of the comprehensive functional skills assessment methodology be the responsibility of a group representing each professional discipline at its highest level of authority. Training in team building is very important for this group as the quality of collaborative, interactive, communication, and decision making that they develop establishes the model for staff and patients and influences all aspects of the model's development and implementation.

Staff education will also include, for all staff, a thorough orientation to the comprehensive functional skills assessment, assessment methods, data analysis, program design procedures, and evaluation.

ASSESSMENT INSTRUMENTS AND METHODS

The number and variety of functional skill assessment instruments in mental health is impressive. Social skills assessment and related training programs have been well documented (Curran & Monti, 1982; Lieberman, 1982; Lieberman, Mueser, & Wallace, 1986; Paul, 1979). Discipline-specific instruments span the areas of self-care, cognition, work skills, task behaviors, sensory motor skills, and many more. Generally these are specific but not comprehensive. Global level of functioning scales are used in many settings (NIMH, 1976), but their lack of specificity is a disadvantage. Anthony and Parkas (1982) identified and categorized some 70 instruments used to assess functional skills and measure outcomes. Only two instruments among these, the New Jersey Level of Function (LOF) and a developing Rhode Island Malfunction Assessment were designated as comprehensive and targeted to an inpatient population.

The New Jersey LOF Scale (Fidler, 1984, New Jersey Level of Functioning, 1976) consists of 43 items aggregated into six subscales: physical functioning, personal care, interpersonal relationships, social acceptability, daily living activities and work skills. One limitation of this instrument is its failure to address the cognitive, affective, or perceptual domains. However, if such assessments are added to those of the scale, it is a workable and comprehensive instrument for assessing functional skills of the adult, nongeriatric patient. The scale, however, is not adequate for assessing the functional skills of the mentally ill elderly or for monitoring changes in their function.

The Parachek Geriatric Rating Scale (Parachek & King, 1976) was designed to assist hospital staff in planning treatment programs for geriatric patients in the state mental hospital. It is a standardized screening device, easily administered within a relatively short period of time. The scale measures three skill categories: physical capabilities, self-care, and social interaction. The descriptive items under each heading are ranged and rated in developmental sequence. Thus, aggregate scores make it possible to separate a population into three levels for program focus. The instrument does provide a rapid and relatively accurate gross profile of the geriatric patient population. Its brevity and lack of breadth, however, limits its usefulness. Such limitations are most evident in the omission of measures of the cognitive and affective domains as well as those aspects of functioning beyond self-care and social interaction.

Level of care assessments are used in many systems to identify the level of care required for nursing home residents. These assessments have been primarily designed for funding purposes and are thus limited to perspectives of nursing care needs. Their usefulness is minimal for planning comprehensive program services or for determining and measuring individual treatment and rehabilitation initiatives.

The Hagedorn Assessment Scale (Hagedorn, 1987) developed and used as part of our project was designed explicitly for the gero-psychiatric patient population to provide indicators for both the design of the program and the formulation of individualized treatment and rehabilitation goals. It is a comprehensive assessment instrument that measures the precursors of performance as well as community living skills. The scale contains 61 items that are categorized into five domains and four community living skills. These include the physical, sensory motor, perceptual, cognitive, affective and interpersonal/social domains, self-care, leisure skills, work-related skills and discharge related behaviors. Additionally the instrument makes it possible to identify those behaviors and/or deficits that are considered critical barriers to discharge. Items identified as critical then become the priority focus for individualized treatment and rehabilitation plans.

This instrument continues to be revised to fine tune its relevance to rehabilitation initiatives for the gero-psychiatric patient. Its reliability and validity needs to be established. We believe, however, that the risks of using a nonstandardized instrument were countered by the fact that ratings of each patient in all instances were the result of interdisciplinary consensus and reflected discipline-specific assessments. Again, it must be emphasized that collaborative decision making is crucial. An instrument is simply a structure for organizing, categorizing and aggregating discipline-specific information and perspectives.

The relevance of a work-related skills category for the geriatric population is frequently questioned. Work and the work ethic have been integral in the daily life of most elderly. Work skills, attitudes, and habits comprise strengths and capacities that enable adaptive responses, sustain health and a sense of personal integrity. The reinforcement of such skills and values is an essential part of any treatment or rehabilitation initiative for this population. Work attitudes and work-related skills are an important variable in the elderly's successful management of community living.

DATA COLLECTION AND ANALYSIS

The tabulation of assessment ratings for each patient provides a numerical score for the patient in each category, that is, each domain and each community living skill. These ratings then form the basis for individualized treatment and rehabilitation goal planning and for monitoring the progress of the patient.

When individual category scores are aggregated for the total patient population, a profile of overall needs and strengths is obtained. These tabulations and the item ratings within each, provide quantitative data of the population with regard to the nature of dysfunction, level of severity, intact strengths, and the number of patients with similar needs, strengths, and problems. This data provides the basis for the design of programs and establishes measurable entry and exit criteria for programs. In addition these criteria serve as reference points for program evaluations, as indicators for appropriate placement of a patient, and for the movement of the patient from one program level to another. The patients' category scores can be aggregated to provide a total assessment score. These total scores are useful primarily when the intent is to create living units of relatively homogeneous levels of functioning.

Our goal was to develop functionally homogeneous living units with unit-specific programs targeted to the special needs and levels of each unit. The total assessment scores were therefore used to determine levels and the cut off score for each level. Some adjustment in this procedure, of course, needed to be made to accommodate the reality of the number of beds on any given unit. For example, our plan called for the creation of a small, transitional living unit to prepare the highest functioning patients for discharge. Because the smallest units contained 22 beds, the 22 highest scoring patients formed this unit. The cut off score being determined by the score of the 22nd patient, that is, 230 points. Out of a possible 305 points, our assessments produced a range from a high score of 297 to a low of 61 points. Nineteen patients were not assessed because of severe and progressive physical and mental deterioration requiring a regimen of almost total nursing care. Using total scores, three major levels of functioning were established. These included: one 22-bed transitional living unit with scores ranging from 297 to 230; two intermediate level units for a total of 56 patients with scores ranging from 229 to 175; four basic-level units for a total of 110 patients, including the 19 nursing care patients and reflecting (exclusive of these 19) a point range of 173 to 61.

Data collection and its analysis makes it possible to functionally describe a patient population, define the required programs and services, and specify the required staff resources. It provides explicit criteria for determining the appropriateness of a given program for a given patient and for measuring outcomes. To facilitate the organization and use of data, two organizing frames or formats were used. The Format for Program Design (see Table 5.1) was developed to identify the points of reference and criteria for the design of programs for each level of functioning. It includes a summary description of the skills-assessment findings, required program services, programming goals, characteristics of the living environment and required staff resources. The Program Protocol (see Table 5.2) is an organizing frame for explicitly defining each program

Table 5.1 Format for Program Design

Points of reference and indicators for the overall design of level-specific programs.

1. *Description of the Patient Population:* A summary of the functional skills-assessment findings. Identification of the nature and level of strengths, deficits, and barriers to discharge which characterize those patients within this grouping. A summary listing of activity interests obtained from an activity interest survey.
2. *Required Program Services:* A listing of specific programs and services that should be provided in order to address the identified needs of this population. These will include health maintenance, leisure programs, as well as remediation programs. Services and programs should be identified by their content and process focus, that is, stress management, group therapy, task-oriented group, prevocational program, leisure interest exploration rather than according to disciplines.
3. *Purpose of Unit Programming:* Identification of the expected placements for patients within the unit; that is, boarding home, group home, nursing home, foster care, family, supervised housing, independent living.
4. *Characteristics of the Daily Living Environment:* Those elements that should characterize the living environment of this unit; that is, the nature of daily routines, schedule requirements, structure, freedom, attitudes, and expectations.
5. *Required Staff Resources:* Identification of the staff expertise, competencies and attitudes that are necessary for the delivery of the required programs. Skills should be referenced to the content and processes identified in the required program; that is, activity group process skills, psychotherapy competencies, restorative nursing skills, and family therapy training.

that has been identified in the Format. The protocol outline that we have used is a revision of an earlier model (Fidler, 1984). It provides for specifying the purpose, rationale, entrance criteria, methodology, and outcome measures of a specific program. A detailed description of these frames and

Table 5.2 Program Protocol

Criteria and outcome measures for a single program or service.

1. *Purpose:* A brief statement that describes the overall goal of the program or service.
2. *Rationale:* A description of the reasons why the program has relevance. The beliefs and constructs that support the validity of the purpose.
3. Anticipated outcomes: Identification of the expected behavioral changes that should result from participation in the program. These should be stated in measurable terms and references to the appropriate functional skill-assessment data.
4. *Entrance criteria:* Identification of the criteria to be used to determine the appropriateness and relevance of the program for a patient. This criteria should include functional skill measures that indicate the level of need and the readiness necessary to enter and benefit from the program or service.
5. *Methodology:* The methods, process, and structure of the program including the frequency, length, and total number of sessions, maximum capacity, location, responsible staff, process methods, and techniques.
6. *Exit criteria:* Those factors and measures used to determine achievement of purpose and expected outcomes. These should be measurable, referenced to anticipated outcomes and to the functional skill-assessment measures.

their use in designing and monitoring programs is addressed in Chapter 6.

MEASURING OUTCOMES

Quality Assurance is the orderly process of examining data that has been collected against established criteria for the purpose of detecting trends and determining the appropriateness of program services. Appropriateness in this sense means proper services provided to proper patients at the proper time of need by qualified, capable staff. (Scalenghe & Duebel, 1987)

A Comprehensive Interdisciplinary Functional Skills Assessment provides a profile of the treatment and rehabilitation needs of a patient population. The Format for Program Design organizes these findings into criteria and indicators for delineating appropriate services, appropriate patients, and appropriately qualified staff. The Program Protocol established measurable indicators for monitoring and evaluating program outcomes, individual patient progress, and the quality and appropriateness of staff performance.

These provide the interdisciplinary team as well as each discipline with ongoing evaluation of program services, enabling early detection of trends that can then be addressed in a timely manner. Individual patient progress is monitored by evaluations from each program in which the patient is partici-

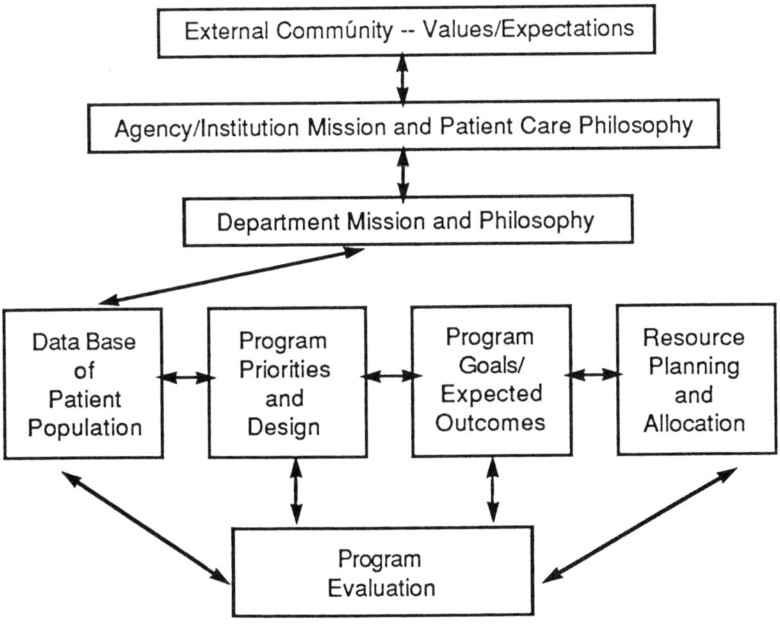

Figure 5.2 Program design process.

pating. Change is regularly reflected and documented in the patient's functional skill assessment.

Accumulation of individual and program evaluation findings over a period of time indicate when there is need for a total analysis of current assessment data and subsequent programmatic changes in the system as a whole. Periodic retabulation and analysis of data is essential for maintaining the integrity of the process. It is a checks and balances system (see Figure 5.2 II, p. 000). The Functional Skills Methodology lends itself readily to computerization, generating an easily managed tracking system for individual patient progress and total program monitoring and evaluation.

REFERENCES

Anthony, W. A., Cohen, M. R., & Cohen, B. F. (1984). Psychiatric rehabilitation. In J. Talbot (Ed.), *The chronic mentally ill: Five years later.* New York: Grune and Stratton.

Anthony, W., & Parkas, M. (1982). A client outcome planning model for assessing psychiatric rehabilitation interventions. *Schizophrenia Bulletin, 8,* 13–38.

Brady, J. P. (1984). Social skills training for psychiatric patients. I: Concepts, methods and clinical results. *American Journal of Psychiatry, 141,* 333–339.

Brady, J. P. (1985). Social skills training for psychiatric patients. II: Clinical outcome studies. *American Journal of Psychiatry, 141,* 491–498.

Brooks, G. (1981). Vocational rehabilitation. In J. A. Talbot (Ed.), *The chronic mentally ill.* New York: Human Sciences Press.

Cohen, B., & Anthony, W. (1984). Functional assessment in pychiatric rehabilitation. In A. Halpern, & M. Fuhrer (Eds.), *Functional assessment in rehabilitation.* Baltimore: Paul Brooks.

Curran, J. P., & Monti, P. M. (Eds.). (1982). *Social skills training: A practical handbook for assessment and treatment.* New York: Guilford.

Fidler, G. S. (1982). The lifestyle performance profile: An organizing frame. In B. J. Hemphill (Ed.), *The Evaluative Process in psychiatric occupational therapy*. Thorofare, NJ: Charles B. Slack.

Fidler, G. S. (1984). *Design of rehabilitation services in psychiatric settings*. Laurel, MD: Ramsco.

Fidler, G. S., and Fidler, J. W. (1978). Doing and becoming: Purposeful action and self actualization, *American Journal of Occupational Therapy, 32,* 305–310.

Fine, S. B. (1980). Psychiatric treatment and rehabilitation: What's in a name? *Journal of National Association of Psychiatric Hospitals, 11,* 8–13.

Gittleman, M., & Freedman, A. M. (1988). Taking issue—treating half of the illness. *American Journal of Psychiatry, 39,* 347.

Goldman, H. H., Gattozzi, A. A., & Taube, C. A. (1981). Defining and counting the chronically mentally ill. *Hospital and Community Psychiatry, 32,* 21–26.

Hagedorn Assessment Scale. (1987). *New Jersey,* Hagedorn Center for Geriatrics, Glen Gardner, NJ: Hagedorn Center for Geriatrics.

Kuehnel, T. G., DeRisi, W. J., Lieberman, R. P., & Mosk, M. (1983). Treatment strategies that promote deinstitutionalization of chronic mental patients. In W. P. Christian, G. T. Hannah, & T. J. Glahn (Eds.), *Deinstitutionalization: Strategies for effective transition of clients to the community*. New York: Plenum Press.

Lieberman, R. P. (1982). Assessment of social skills. *Schizophrenia Bulletin, 8,* 62–83.

Lieberman, R. P., Mueser, K. T., and Wallace, C. J. (1986). Social skills training for schizophrenic individuals at risk for relapse. *American Journal of Psychiatry, 143,* 523–526.

Minkoff, K. (1987). Beyond deinstitutionalization: New ideology for the postinstitutional era. *Hospital and Community Psychiatry, 38,* 945–950.

National Institutes of Mental Health. (1976). *A client-oriented system of mental health service delivery and program management: A workbook and guide*. Publication No. (ADM) 80–307, Superintendent of Documents, Series FN No. 4. Washington, DC: U.S. Government Printing Office.

New Jersey Division of Mental Health and Hospitals, Bureau of Standards. (1976). *Level of Functioning Assessment*. Princeton, NJ.

Parachek, J. F., & King, L. J. (1976). *Parachek Geriatric Rating Scale*. Scottsdale, AZ: Greenroom Publications.

Paul, G. L., & Lentz, R. J. (1977). *Psychosocial treatment for chronic mental patients: Milieu versus social learning programs*. Cambridge, MA: Harvard University Press.

Paul, G. L. (1979). New assessment systems for residential treatment, management, research and evaluation: A symposium. *Journal of Behavioral Assessment, 1*, 181–184.

Scalenghe, R. W., & Deubel, M. (1987). Making the transition: hospital based psychiatric services and the AMH. Chicago IL: Joint Commission on Accreditation of Hospitals.

6 Program Planning

The design of a comprehensive treatment and rehabilitation program is an interdisciplinary endeavor. Each discipline applies its specific expertise, while interacting and planning with other disciplines around goals with a common focus. The end product is expected to be an integrated and comprehensive set of programs discernibly relevant to the specific needs of a given population.

The basic orientation for the design of programs should include two interrelated components. These can be broadly categorized as (1) those services and programs that are concerned with the remediation of dysfunction and the treatment of illness and, (2) those programs that encourage and support healthy behaviors, making it possible for patients to use and refine individual abilities, strengths, and interests, and thus enhance the quality of their lives. The Comprehensive Functional Skills Assessment makes it possible to more explicitly specify and measure such purposes. It identifies the abilities and dysfunctions of a population and enables definition of those programs and services that are required to address identified problems. For example, examination of our functional skills assessment data revealed that in the Interpersonal/Social Domain, 51 patients scored in the bottom half of this scale. Therefore some rather fundamental social/interpersonal skill learning and practice was required for these 51 patients. Among these, 29 scored in the bottom quarter of the scale. An item analysis showed that these 29 patients required programming to address isolation, withdrawn and unresponsive behaviors, and fearfulness of others. In contrast, there were 20 other patients whose relatively high ratings indicated that their programs should provide opportunity to use and reinforce their social engagement interests and skills. In addition, the item analysis revealed the need for a program focus on their problems of managing conflict, developing self-advocacy skills, and increasing awareness of the needs and feelings of others.

In the cognitive domain our data analysis reflected the need for programming to address critical deficits in orientation, judgment, concentration, and sequencing for 19 patients. Additionally, there were 22 patients who scored in the upper level of this scale with principal strengths in concentration, memory, recall and goal-directed behaviors. Deficit areas were shown as lack of awareness of their own problems, faulty cause-and-effect reasoning and poor problem-solving skills. Thus, the program priority in this area and the context in which such groups would function (i.e. strengths), was evident for these 22 patients.

Analysis of scores in the affective domain revealed that 24 patients evidenced severe problems relative to motivation, flat affect, unresponsive and/or inappropriate behaviors. Thus, a program focus to address problems of these 24 patients was clearly identified. Data analysis also showed that there were 12 patients who scored in the top 25% of this domain. An item analysis indicated a need for programs that would sustain and reinforce the high motivation of these patients by helping them learn more effective ways of coping with perceived stress and managing frustration.

ORGANIZING DATA: A FORMAT FOR PROGRAM PLANNING

From these brief examples, one can see how the focus for programs, the level of that focus, as well as the number of patients within each group begins to emerge. A procedure for organizing data is an important first step. The Format for Program Planning (see Table 5.1 on p. 83) was developed as a frame for organizing data into criteria and guidelines for program planning and services. It includes the following elements.

1. *A summary description of the patient population.* This is a summary of the functional skills-assessment findings. Identification of the nature and level of strengths, deficits, and barriers to discharge that characterize those patients within this grouping. A summary listing of activity interests is obtained from an activity-interest survey.

2. *Required program services.* This is a listing of those programs and services that should be provided in view of the identified needs of this population. These will include health-maintaining leisure programs as well as remediation programs. The importance of recognizing and enabling patients to use their strengths and interests cannot be over emphasized. Remediation programs must always be designed within the context of the capabilities of the patient. However, the other critical dimension concerns a focus on the design of those programs that are required in order for the patient to use and reinforce strengths, capacities, and interests. Work and volunteer service opportunities are one example as are those activities associated with leisure and recreation. Services and programs should be identified by their content and process focus, for example, stress management, group therapy, task-oriented groups, prevocational activities, leisure exploration, and the like, rather than according to disciplines. The identification of the content focus of a program in preference to a focus on disciplines is an important variable in defining and determining needed resources. All too frequently, programs are designed around staff rather than patient needs. Staffing is frequently determined by a discipline's perceived need or bias in contrast to an objective consideration of the staff skills and expertise that are

needed. Patient programs thus get shaped by territorial rights and/or the expedient role blurring philosophy that says "Most anyone can do most anything, especially if 'I' oversee the doing." The explicit delineation of required program services, based on functional skills-assessment data, does bring some objectivity to the process of establishing program priorities.

3. *Purpose of unit programming.* The identification of the expected discharge placement of patients, for example boarding home, group home, nursing home, foster care, family, supervised housing, independent living. This is a critical consideration in planning programs and in the placement of a patient in a given program. The kind and level of skills and behaviors that the patient will need to learn or redevelop is determined by the kind of environment in which that patient will be living. We know this in fact, but the knowing seems to get lost in program planning or in its implementation. Menu planning, for example, in preparation for life in a boarding home or community leisure exploration for patients going to a nursing home are at the very least dishonest. The significance of considering the discharge placement of the patient should by no means preclude opportunities and incentives to maximize the patient's potential. However, when a plateau is reached and when an appropriate discharge placement is evident, the program priority for the patient must be preparation to enter and to satisfyingly adapt to that environment.

4. *Characteristics of the daily environment:* Specification of those elements which, given the purpose of the unit and the functional level of patients, should characterize the living environment. This will include the physical characteristics, the principal elements of daily routine and schedule requirements; the way the unit should operate, for example the nature and kind of structure and freedom; principle expectations and requirements for patient and staff behaviors and significant staff attitudes. The environment is a dynamic in its own right. Physical elements such as light, color, sound, temperature, furnishings and their arrangement, the nature of the overall operation of a unit or floor, influence, reflect, and reinforce staff and patient attitudes, behaviors, and expectations. The nature of an environment does indeed have an impact on program outcomes. Describing the essential characteristics of a given environment is therefore an important part of program planning.

5. *Required staff resources.* Identification of the staff expertise, competencies and attitudes that are necessary for the delivery of the

required programs. Necessary skills and expertise should again be referenced to the program content and processes that have been identified in the Required Program Services. These will include for example, activity group process skills, psychotherapy competencies, group therapy skills, training skills in personal hygiene and grooming, community ADL programming expertise. Staff attitudes and interests would address for example, values and beliefs regarding staff responsibility, patient decision making and responsibility, consistent orderly operations, patient autonomy and the like.

APPLICATION OF THE FORMAT

The following examples will show how the Format for Program Planning was used to develop criteria and guidelines for programs and services in two of our patient units. The Transitional Living Unit was a 22-bed unit housing the highest functioning patients. Total functional skills-assessment ratings for this group ranged from a high of 297, out of a possible 305 points, to a low of 230. In addition to this unit, there were three intermediate units with functional skills-assessment ratings ranging from 229 to 175 points and three basic living units with patients rated from a high of 173 to 61 points. The basic unit, with scores ranging from a high of 139 points to a low of 112, will be used as an example to contrast with the Transitional unit. This basic level unit had a bed capacity of 33.

Transitional Living Unit

1. Summary Description of the Patient Population
   a. No significant health problems. All functions within the physical, sensory-motor domains are within normal limits for this age group. Physical stamina is rated low (19 patients).
   b. Conditional relationships with peers, family, and staff (10 patients). Limited repertoire of interpersonal coping skills, especially in relation to: appropriate assertiveness, self-advocacy and independence (22 patients); sensitivity to needs and feelings of others (18 patients); handling conflicts,

compromising, negotiating (22 patients); taking the social initiative required to meet personal needs and prevent isolation (20 patients).

   c. Affect is generally appropriate. Decompensates, demonstrates high anxiety in response to change, increased expectations, frustration and other perceived stressors (22 patients).
   d. Good memory, recall, reality orientation, and temporal adaptation (19 patients). Lacks awareness of own problems (16 patients); has realistic view of self, others and the environment (21 patients); poor problem solving skills (18 patients); poor judgment (18 patients).
   e. Independent in personal hygiene, dressing, grooming, care of own living space and personal possessions (22 patients). Lack of adequate self-care skills for community living related to money management, banking, shopping, travel, meal preparation, self-medication, health care (22 patients);
   f. Good work-related skills, attitudes, and habits but needs to apply these in more normalized settings (20 patients).
   g. Appropriate and adequate leisure interests but requires assistance to manage free time and independently pursue activities both in the local community and on grounds (16 patients).
   h. Views the community with fear and apprehension. Unaware of community resources, services, or lifestyles (19 patients).
   i. Chronic institutional dependency (19 patients).

2. Required Program Services
   a. Community ADL Skills Development: small groups with a focus on developing independent skills related to: budgeting, banking, clothing care, shopping, self-medication, health care, meal planning and preparation, basic reading, and computation skills.
   b. Verbal and Task-Oriented Groups for learning and practice related to: assertion and self-advocacy; self-awareness; negotiating and compromising skills; managing stress; communicating and relating to others: making friends, establishing contact, learning about others; problem solving, learning cause and effect, reasoning; managing free time; family relationships; family counseling.
   c. Work and Work-Related Activities: work and volunteer service opportunities within the institution and in the local

community to use and reinforce strengths and interests, these to include but not necessarily be limited to the following opportunities:

food services	typist
cashier	receptionist
store clerk	mail delivery/messenger service
maintenance: services	cottage industries
housekeeping services	green thumb
greenhouse	meals on wheels
patient volunteer services	
local church volunteer groups	

d. Leisure activities in the local community and on grounds to address the skills and principal interests of the patients that have been identified in the functional skills assessment and the Activity Interest Survey. These include music listening and concerts, group singing, play acting, card games, plant care and gardening, sightseeing trips, writing, newspaper, sports events, socials, cooking, and needlecrafts.

e. Daily Therapeutic Community meetings.

3. Purpose of Unit Programming

The purpose of this unit was to prepare the patient for community living in one of the following environments: boarding home, group home, supervised housing, shared apartment, foster home or one's family.

To achieve this purpose, the principal objectives of programming on the unit were to enable the patient to: increase his/her independence; diminish reliance on staff; learn shared responsibility and collaborative skills; develop community-living skills sufficient to satisfactorily sustain self in the appropriate community environment; diminish anxiety and fears about leaving the institution.

4. Characteristics of the Daily Environment

a. The total environment will: respect and expect adult behaviors; expect that patients are responsible for their daily routines, for the management of their time, their schedules and behaviors; expect that patients take responsibility for maintaining their living units; provide realistic, validating, cause and effect feedback; allow learning through trial and error; reflect the belief that patients can make valid decisions regarding their own lives; expect a balance of participation among work, leisure pursuit, and self-maintenance activities; provide for personal time and reflection as well as social engagement; offer comfortable, efficient, attractive working and socializing settings; expect effective, ongoing daily staff communication and sharing over 24-hour periods; expect patients to be actively involved in planning their own recreational programs; approximate the behavioral expectations and lifestyles characteristics of the outside community; expect participation of all patients and all staff in the daily therapeutic community meetings and processes; expect that the role of staff is more that of mentor, counselor, and teacher than caregiver, monitor, or director.

b. Structure and schedule expectations: Each patient is expected to work and/or provide volunteer services for no less than ten hours a week. Treatment and rehabilitation programs are given top priority during morning and early afternoon hours, Monday through Friday, for a total of no less than three hours per day. Recreational activities and programs both on grounds and in the community are scheduled for late afternoons, evenings, weekends, and holidays. Team and staff meetings are scheduled so as not to interrupt or compete with patient treatment or rehabilitation programs. Team meetings are scheduled at times that make it possible for evening staff to participate. Patients weekend activities and time schedules approximate those of the outside community.

5. Required Staff Resources
   a. Staff attitudes and values should include: belief in the value to the patient of living outside of the institution; the willingness to learn and try out a different approach to patient treatment and management; comfort with collective patient decision making; belief that individuals will rise to meet the expectations that others have for them; belief that the patient is capable of responsible, adult behaviors; a healthy respect for individual autonomy; belief in the efficacy of group process and open communication, comfort with each.
   b. Necessary staff skills and expertise: training and experience in two or more of the following: community ADL skill development; work programs; health education, health monitoring, and self-medication programs; verbal group process; group psychotherapy; family therapy and counse-

ling; psychoeducation programs; cognitive therapy; task-oriented group process; activity group process; activity and leisure programs; community liaison and community services; discharge planning and placement;

The staff mix and numbers will be computed on the basis that (1) the required programs will serve all 22 patients and, (2) remedial programs will be scheduled no less than three times a week; (3) medical services and monitoring will be provided by means of part-time consultation. The need for nursing services per se will be quite minimal.

The Basic Unit

1. Summary Description of the Patient Population
   a. Physical Domain: no significant health problems; diminished visual and auditory functions associated with aging but no severe disability; unclear speech with inappropriate rate and tone (17 patients); continence problems requiring continual reminders and assistance (17 patients); poor tolerance for moderate physical exertion (17 patients); slow, shuffling, unsteady gait (20 patients).
   b. Sensory-Motor Perceptual Domain: poor gross motor coordination, poor balance and nonintegrated movements (20 patients); inadequate eye-hand coordination (19 patients); hallucinations interfere with function (15 patients).
   c. Cognitive Domain: attention span and concentration are sufficient only for very short-term tasks or activities (17 patients); lack of goal-directed behaviors (19 patients); poor judgment jeopardizing safety (29 patients); inability to recognize causal relationships (29 patients); inability to manage illogical, incoherent thinking (22 patients).
   d. Affective Domain: affect inappropriate (24 patients); inability to tolerate frustration or disappointment (26 patients); lack of a sense of pleasure or satisfaction (15 patients); lethargic, unresponsive behaviors, lack of motivation (18 patients).
   e. Interpersonal Social Skills Domain: communication and interpersonal functioning are characterized by unresponsive or irrelevant behaviors (15 patients); inability to form relationships with peers (29 patients); discomfort in group situations (20 patients); unacceptable, inappropriate behavior

that requires substantial external limits and control (18 patients).

f. Self-Care and Maintenance: independent personal hygiene and grooming care (10 patients); self-care requires regular verbal assistance (11 patients); self-care requires extensive verbal reminders and physical assistance (12 patients); unsafe, socially unacceptable eating patterns and habits (14 patients); requires considerable assistance to care for own living area (23 patients); ability to care for own living area with minimal assistance (10 patients).

g. Leisure Skills: inability to pursue leisure activities without extensive encouragement and assistance (24 patients); inability to identify interests (18 patients); lack of an expression of pleasure with leisure activities (22 patients). The levels of functioning of these patients makes it difficult to discern leisure interests or previous leisure skills. Although the activity interest survey was completed with the patients, it is especially difficult to distinguish a genuine interest on the part of the patient from a concern with pleasing staff.

h. Work/Work-Related Skills: this category is not relevant to this patient population at this time. The level of skills required is beyond the present capacity of the patients. Out of a possible score of 35 points in this area, the average score was 7. More fundamental functions and behaviors must be addressed before the patient can be expected to respond to the functional expectations identified in this category.

2. Required Program Services

a. Individual and small group program for articulation, vocalization, hearing and comprehending others, basic communication skills; bowel and bladder-training programs; gross motor exercise and mobility training.

b. Activities promoting sensory awareness and perceptual integration. small groups to focus on proprioceptive facilitation, sensory stimulation, eye tracking, postural flexibility, space and form perception, directionality, figure–ground awareness, laterality, and body-image activities, breathing and relaxation techniques.

c. Cognitive stimulation and functioning; small task-oriented groups and organized structural games focused on: stimulating cognitive processes; organizing thought; providing cues for sequencing; reality orientation; causal awareness; stimulation of memory and recall.

d. Interpersonal and Social Skill Learning; small circle and group games and activities that provide: parallel and casual encounters; awareness and recognition of others; ensured success and recognition of achievement; response to others; group sharing.

e. Personal Hygiene: dressing and grooming programs at the basic level (I) and at the more advanced level (II); programs to promote appropriate eating habits and patterns; small group and individualized programs for learning to care for own living area with increased responsibility.

A variety of leisure activity focused on the interests identified by the patients and offered so as to maximize gross motor activity, social and interpersonal awareness, the stimulation of all senses and most especially on having fun.

3. Purpose of Unit Programming

The purpose of the unit was to enable the patient to: eliminate disruptive or inappropriate behavior that prevents entry into a community-based nursing home; develop self-care skills in order to enhance one's own sense of autonomy and to be acceptable in a nursing-home environment; develop social, interpersonal, and leisure skills to maximize the quality of life; or, improve functioning so as to meet the entrance requirements of the intermediate unit; to provide a human and nonhuman environment that is consistent, predictable, clarifying and responsive; onc that enables continuous practice and a balanced, normalizing lifestyle.

4. Characteristics of the Daily Environment

a. The total environment will: provide a high degree of structure, clear and consistent organization and scheduling; reflect an appreciation for repetition and practice; expect that functional improvement is possible; reflect a respect for the importance of a sense of autonomy; provide clear standards and expectations for behavior; value and validate the adult in each person; provide support and positive reinforcement for abilities and achievements; reflect a tolerance for error without threatening the integrity of the person; provide cues that facilitate functioning; stimulate all senses.

b. Structure and schedule expectations: each patient will have his/her own individual schedule; all interdisciplinary staff and team meetings will take place after 2:30 P.M.; daily community meetings will be held just prior to lunch; toileting and personal hygiene programs for levels I and II will occur prior to breakfast; continence programs are in operation 24 hours a day; a 30-minute rest period is scheduled immediately after lunch; all patients will take their meals in the central dining room unless this is not possible because of illness; eating habits and behavior programs will occur in the dining room during meal times; treatment and rehabilitation groups are scheduled for 40 minutes and are held mid-morning and early afternoon Monday through Friday.

There are formalized consistent procedures for communication between day, evening, night, and weekend staff; leisure activities are scheduled for late afternoon, early evening, weekends, and holidays; each patient is assigned to a line nursing care staff who functions as mentor for that patient.

5. Required Staff Resources
   a. Staff attitudes and values: a respect and appreciation for a high degree of structure, clear and consistent organization and repetition; ability to gain satisfaction from cumulative small gains over a prolonged period of time; recognition and belief in the importance of consistent and repetitive practice; ability to supportively and caringly engage with patients at this level of dysfunction; expectations that functional improvement is possible; capacity to support the purposes of this unit and the characteristics of its environment;
   b. Necessary staff skills and expertise, training and experience in two or more of the following: nonverbal activity group process; programs focused on: sensory stimulation; body response and integrated movements; perceptual integration; basic interpersonal and social skill development; continence training; physical restoration; personal hygiene, dressing, and grooming; basic communication skills; articulation, vocalization, hearing and responding; leisure programming for basic level of functioning patients; environmental structuring with basic level population; behavior modification techniques.

Staff mix and numbers will be based on the number of patients for whom programs will be needed as specified in the summary of the patient population.

ESTABLISHING PROGRAM CRITERIA

The Program Protocol

The next critical step in program planning is to set measurable standards for each program that will be offered at each level. The Program Protocol (see Table 5.2 on p. 84) is an organizing frame for explicitly defining measurable criteria for a given treatment or rehabilitation intervention. As such it provides outcome measures for individual patient progress as well as criteria for evaluating the appropriateness and effectiveness of a given program. This document includes the following elements:

1. *Purpose:* A brief statement that describes the overall goal of the program or service.
2. *Rationale:* A description of the reasons why the program has relevance. The beliefs and constructs that support the validity of the purpose.
3. *Anticipated Outcomes:* Identification of expected behavioral changes, which should result from participation in the program, stated in measurable terms and referenced to the appropriate functional skill assessment data.
4. *Entrance Criteria:* Identification of the established criteria to be used to determine the appropriateness and relevance of the program for a given patient. Functional skill measures that indicate the level of need and readiness necessary to enter and benefit from the program.
5. *Methodology:* The methods, process and structure of the program including the frequency, length, and total number of sessions, maximum capacity, location, responsible staff, methods and process technique.

6. *Exit Criteria:* Those factors and measures used to determine exit from the program. These should be measurable, referenced to anticipated outcomes and functional skills—assessment measures.

The involvement of staff in the development of program protocols is an excellent learning experience. It provides practice in the ever elusive skill of writing measurable objectives. Even more important, the development of protocols helps staff to clarify what it is they do, why they do it, and how they can judge the effectiveness of their services. Finally, the protocols are a resource and guide to treatment teams in making decisions about referrals to programs and ensuring, insofar as possible, the most relevant utilization of existing resources for the patient.

Examples of how the functional skills assessment data can be used to establish program criteria are as follows.

Program Protocol

Group Living Skills Unit

Community Resources Exploration Group

Purpose To provide opportunities for visits to community placement sites, to become familiar with living alternatives in the community and thus to reduce the fear and anxiety associated with discharge.

Rationale Long-term institutionalization results in prolonged estrangement from community life. Fear of what is now the unknown, the recall of trauma and problems of coping with previous institutional settings, generate inordinate anxiety and resistance to leaving the secure, predictable environment of the Center. Becoming aware of alternatives, seeing what life is like on the outside, discovering that many who are now living in the community once experienced the same anxiety, sharing impressions and doubts with understanding peers and staff, are the first steps in bridging the unknown, reducing fears, and beginning to plan for discharge.

Anticipated Outcomes

- Awareness of the different characteristics of community-living environments.
- Identification of the positive aspects of living in such environments.
- Reduction in the frequency and intensity of negative reactions to life outside.
- Expression of some preference for a particular setting.
- Open discussion with peers and staff regarding possible community living.
- Expression of a willingness to begin work on a discharge plan.
- Improved assessment scores in Discharge-Related Behaviors Category.

Entrance Criteria

- Placement in Group Living Skills Program.
- Absence of a family or the impossibility of placement with the natural family.
- Evidence of fear and resistance to discharge.
- Except for resistance factor, assessment data indicates readiness for discharge to: group home, boarding home, foster home, senior citizen residence, shared apartment.
- Assessment scores on Discharge-Related Behaviors are: items 1 through 3, 4 or above, item 2 a score of 5, item 4, 3 or below.

Methodology

- Sessions: 4 hours weekly for 8 weeks
- Group Capacity: eight
- Location: Fairweather House
- Process: The group will meet to plan for and visit those community placements available to patients from the Center. These will include group homes, boarding homes, foster homes, senior citizen residences and shared apartments. Following each visit

the group will share impressions, discuss the positive and negative aspects of the setting and its potential as a living arrangement for individual members.

Exit Criteria

One or more of the following:

- A score of 4 or above on item 4, Category IV.
- Consistent pattern of more positive than negative opinions regarding life in the community.
- Expression of a community placement preference.
- Expressed interest in working an a discharge plan.
- Attends fewer that 5 sessions.
- Does not participate in planning or discussions.
- Behavior is inappropriate and disruptive.
- Refuses to continue.

Program Protocol

Intermediate Level

Relating to Others Group I

Purpose To learn and practice, within a group context, ways of:

- initiating contact with others
- discovering the interests and preferences of others
- expressing personal preferences and interests
- handling disagreement

Rationale Withdrawal and isolation from others are behaviors frequently related to a chronic mental illness, prolonged hospitalization, and is compounded by diminishing capacities related to aging. Limited incentive and opportunities to establish reciprocal relationships diminishes the use of interpersonal skills and, over time, results in the loss of such skills and their intrinsic motivations. Relatedness to others is a basic human need. It is essential to a state of health and life satisfaction. Some level of tolerance and acceptance of another is critical to living with others.

Anticipated Outcomes

- Increased frequency of contact with others
- Awareness of similarities and differences between self and others
- Expressed interest in and concern for another
- Behaviors that help others become part of a group or endeavor
- Expressed satisfaction in relating to others
- Tolerance for negotiating disagreement
- Improved assessment scores in the interpersonal/social domain

Entrance Criteria

- Evidence of difficulty relating to others with significant problems in awareness of others, forming peer relationships and comfort in a group.
- A score of 3 or below on all items in the Interpersonal/Social Domain except: a score below 3 on items 27, 30, 33, and 35. The physical, cognitive, and perceptual ability to cope with the content and process of this group. Thus a score of 3 or above in the following: A—items 2 and 5; B—item 9; C—items 11, 13, 17 and 20; D—item 26. Personal hygiene and grooming—a score of 3 or above.

Methodology

- Sessions: 1 hour, 3 times a week for 8 weeks
- Group Capacity: 8
- Process: A combination of educational and experiential approaches will be used for each session. These will include a brief lecture or presentation of a topic related to the purpose of the group followed by a role play and practice component relevant to the content, and finally a discussion of the lecture material and experiences of the session.

Exit Criteria

One or more of the following:

- A score of 3 or above on items 27, 30, 33, and 35 in the Interpersonal/Social Domain.
- Increased frequency of initiating and sustaining contact with others.
- Improved scores in two or more of the following items in the Interpersonal/Social Domain—28, 29, 31, 32, 34.

- Attendance at fewer than 5 sessions.
- Persistent lack of participation in the experiential or discussion phases of most sessions.
- Refusal to attend.

Program Protocol

Basic Level

Exercise/Relaxation Group I

Purpose To provide a range of gross motor activities to stimulate awareness, improve the organization of sensory and proprioceptive input, of cognitive and affective responses in order to enhance awareness and appropriateness of response to external events.

Rationale Prolonged mental illness and diminished sensory capacities associated with aging generate problems in receiving, organizing, and interpreting messages from the outside world and from one's own body. The result is a diminished or distorted perception of what is going on and a corresponding paucity of response, or overreaction and/or inappropriate behavior. Selected sequential sensory-motor activities, offered in an environment that controls against sensory overload can elicit attention and improve the ability to organize and more accurately interpret messages. The capacity for appropriate and productive response to treatment and rehabilitation opportunities is thus enhanced.

Anticipated Outcomes
- Increased attention to events in the immediate environment.
- Reduced preoccupation with hallucinations and/or reduction of inappropriate responses.
- Improved response and participation.
- Increased attention span.
- Demonstrated awareness of others.
- More frequent, appropriate response to others.
- Improved scores in the sensory-motor, cognitive, affective, and interpersonal social domains.

Entrance Criteria

- A combined score within the range of 44 to 73 points in the sensory-motor, cognitive, affective, and interpersonal social domains.
- Assessments reflecting serious problems in three or more of the following: isolated-unresponsive behavior, flat and/or inappropriate affect, preoccupation with hallucinations, inappropriate behaviors, postural rigidity, poor muscle tone and coordination, and lack of motivation.

Methodology

- Sessions: 30 minutes, 5 times a week
- Group Capacity: 10
- Location: Small gym
- Process: This is an open, ongoing group. New patients will be added as vacancies occur. The patient is retained in the group until maximum benefit is achieved as measured by exit criteria and anticipated outcomes—or patient is terminated because of lack of participation as specified in the exit criteria. Patients will be involved in a series of sequential gross motor activities that will focus on bodily response, postural flexibility, muscle tone and physical endurance, space and form perception, left–right directionality, figure–ground awareness, integration of both sides of the body, body image, building, and relaxation.

Exit Criteria

- Improved scores in the sensory-motor, cognitive, affective and interpersonal/social domains reflecting a combined total score of 74 points or above.
- Significant improvements in responsiveness, postural flexibility, affect, and motivation.
- Physical and/or mental deterioration that has made active participation impossible.
- Lack of participation or failure to attend sessions for 10 consecutive sessions.

INDIVIDUALIZING PROGRAMS

The comprehensive functional-skills assessment yields a numerical rating for each patient in each domain and each community-living skills category. These ratings form the basis for individualized treatment and rehabilitation goal setting. They also serve as indicators and monitors of patient progress. When the rating scale provides for identification of those dysfunctions that are considered critical to discharge, these become the priority focus for individualized goals. The following examples will illustrate these points.

EDWARD R.

A review of ER's updated functional skills assessment indicated that he was sustaining an adequate level of functioning except in two areas. He was rated at level II on items 23 and 24 in the affective domain and an even lower score of 1 on item 56 in the work-skills category. The affective domain ratings noted serious problems in managing stress and coping with disappointment and frustration. His low frustration tolerance was evident for example in his handling delays in the cafeteria line, by resorting to angry disruptive outbursts. Similar behavior occurred in other settings but was most critical in his otherwise commendable functioning in the work shop. He was unable to sustain work when he was frustrated and because of his low frustration tolerance, disruption was all too frequent.

These behaviors were considered critical as ER would be living in a supervised housing program and would work in the community sheltered workshop. The patient and the treatment team agree that his low frustration tolerance is a real barrier to his discharge.

Problems

1. A score of 2 on items 23 and 24, Affective Domain:
   - ineffective coping with perceived stressful situation
   - intolerance of disappointment or frustration.
2. A score of 1 on item 56, Work-Related Skills:
   - unable to sustain work effort when frustrated.

Strengths

1. Affective Domain item 26, score of 5, patient is motivated to pursue therapeutic opportunities.

2. Work-Related Skills category:
   - item 51, score of 5, values work
   - item 52, score of 4, has specific work interests
   - item 54, score of 4, responsible work habits

Long-Term Goal

- Improved score on items 23, 24, and 56 by at least one point.
- A score of 4 on item 24 before ER can be discharged to the supervised housing program

Short-Term Goal

- Reduce the frequency of maladaptive response to frustration.

Objectives

1. Patient will remain in the workshop for three consecutive work sessions within the next two weeks.
2. Patient will tell the supervisor on at least two occasions when he is beginning to feel upset.
3. Patient will attend the intermediate level group on managing stress.

Intervention Strategies

1. Workshop supervisor will reduce task requirements to no more than a three-step process.
2. Supervisor will support patient in verbalizing his discomfort and will provide an appropriate relief when stress is perceived.
3. Group on managing stress will focus on helping the patient develop alternative patterns for managing his frustration.

SARA M.

A review of SM's functional skills assessment revealed a significant problem in two related aspects of behavior. She was given a rating of 2 on item 9 in the Sensory-Motor/Perceptual Domain and a significantly low score of 1 on item 47 in the Leisure Skills Category. These ratings indicated serious problems related to her management of hallucinations and her pursuit of leisure interests. Although SM has described a number of leisure interests, she has regularly refused to participate in scheduled evening or weekend activities, labeling these as "child's play."

It is evident that SM does hallucinate but this has not interfered with functioning in her part-time job assignment as typist/receptionist, in her work with the newspaper group, or in her responsibilities as patient council secretary. However, when she is inactive such as during evening hours, she becomes increasingly preoccupied with the voices, agitated, verbally abusive and threatening to patients, creating turmoil and a management problem in the day room. It was further noted that her rating was high in relationships with staff and low in the ability to relate to peers.

These problems are critical as plans are underway for SM to enter a group home and be employed part time as receptionist/typist at the local senior citizen center.

Problems

1. A score of 2, item 9, Sensory-Motor/Perceptual Domain: ineffective management of hallucinations.
2. A score of 1, item 47, Leisure Skills Category—does not pursue leisure interests during free time.

Strengths

Cognitive domain item 18, score of 4, patient can solve problems as they arise. Item 19, score of 5, patient is goal directed.

Interpersonal Domain: item 32, score of 4, patient forms and maintains good relationship with staff.

Work-Related Skills: item 51, score of 5, patient views work as important and fulfilling; item 52, score of 4, has specific work interests; and item 54, score of 5, responsible work habits.

Long-Term Goals

1. Improved score on items 9 and 47 to at least a rating of 3.
2. A score of 4 before SM can enter the group home project.

Short-Term Goals

1. SM will increase and sustain her leisure activity during evening hours.
2. SM will manage her hallucinations so that her behavior is not disruptive to others.

Objectives

SM will:

1. Select one of her expressed leisure interests.
2. Work with the Recreational Therapist (RT) in planning and carrying out the activity.
3. Carry out her planned choice on at least two evenings during the week for the next two weeks.
4. See Dr. F one time a week for the next ten weeks for the purpose of managing her hallucinations.
5. Join the advanced level community leisure resources group.

Intervention Strategies

The recreational therapist will:

1. Verify and reinforce SM's strengths.
2. Assist SM in critically assessing her interests and skills.
3. Work toward SM's pursuit of relevant, realistic leisure patterns and activities.
4. Support SM's involvement in the Community Leisure Resource Group.

The Community Leisure Resource Group will focus on SM's exploration and use of community resources.

Dr. F will use counseling and psychoeducation as principal strategies.

PATIENT CASE MONITORING AND PROGRAM EVALUATION

In Chapter 5 we talked about quality assurance standards and how the segments of a functional skills-assessment methodology generated a checks and balance system for ensuring proper services to proper patients at the proper time of need by properly qualified staff. The efficacy of any program design is measured by (1) its effect on the patient and (2) the degree of relevance of the program to patient needs. The Functional Skills Assessment, the Format for Program Planning, and the Program Protocol each address aspects of these criteria.

It is essential that program planning include those monitoring and evaluative measures that will be used to determine program validity. It has been argued that these measures should be incorporated into the Format for Program Planning. However, because measures are the same for all programs and services, it seems reasonable to incorporate them in the overall quality assurance program standards of each relevant department and/or discipline.

Patient Care Monitoring comprises those activities and procedures that are used to track patient progress, the level of the patient's program participation, response to and overall course of treatment and rehabilitation. Procedures include:

1. Record of attendance with reasons for absences.
2. Routine monitoring and evaluation of those behaviors specified in the anticipated outcomes and exit criteria of each program/service in which the patient is involved.
3. Monthly documentation of progress in the medical record based on above criteria.
4. A final summary when the patient exits a program that summarizes progress by recording achievement or limitations relative to program-anticipated outcomes and exit criteria.

Program Evaluation involves those steps that will be taken to collect, aggregate, and analyze patient care monitoring data and to determine the impact of programs in relation to patients and their needs. This analysis of data should attempt to determine achievement of anticipated outcomes, the appropriateness of entrance and exit criteria, and the effectiveness of methodology and duration of the program. Data collection for each program or service should include:

- attendance records with number of absences and reasons why absent
- total number of patients placed on entry waiting list
- total number of unfilled slots
- total number of referrals
- number and kind of inappropriate referrals

- number and percentage of patients successfully achieving anticipated outcomes
- number and percentage of patients failing to achieve anticipated outcomes
- number and percentage of patients achieving anticipated outcomes before specified time limit of group sessions
- analysis of improved/unimproved scores
- analysis of staff expertise required and staff actually used.

In summary, the design and evaluation of comprehensive programs is, as we stated at the beginning of this chapter, an interdisciplinary, patient-focused effort. It is as much the result of collaborative dialogue as is the comprehensive functional skills assessment, the therapeutic community, and the creation of a responsive, clarifying environment. Program planning is one part, one unit of a whole. In the last analysis its efficacy will be known by the nature of the interactional processes among all units of the system.

SUGGESTED READINGS

Anthony, W. A. (1981). *Principles of psychiatric rehabilitation.* Baltimore: University Park Press.

Anthony W., Cohen, M., & Cohen, B. (1984). *The philosophy, treatment process and principles of the psychiatric rehabilitation approach.* Center for Rehabilitation Research and Training, Boston University, Boston, MA.

Anthony, W. A., Cohen, M. R., & Cohen, B. F. (1984). In J. Talbot (Ed.), *Psychiatric rehabilitation in the chronic mentally ill: Five years later.* New York: Grune and Stratton.

Christian, W. P., Hannah, G. T., & Glahn, T. J. (Eds.) (1983). *Deinstitutionalization: Strategies for effective transition of clients to the community.* New York: Plenum Press.

Curran, J. P., & Monti, P. M. (Ed.) (1982). *Social skills training: A practical handbook for assessment and treatment.* New York: Guilford.

Dougherty, P. M., & Radonski, M. V. (1987). *The cognitive rehabilitation workbook.* Rockville, MD: Aspen.

Fairweather, G. W. (1981). *The Fairweather lodge: A twenty-five year retrospective.* San Francisco: Jossey-Bass.

Fairweather, G. W., Sanders, G. H., Gessler, D. L., & Maynard, H. (1969). *Community life for the mentally ill.* Chicago: Aldine Publishing.

Fidler, G. S. (1984). *Design of rehabilitation services in psychiatric hospital settings.* Laurel, MD: Ramsco.

Fine, S. B. (1980). Psychiatric treatment and rehabilitation: What's in a Name? *Journal of National Association of Psychiatric Hospitals, 11*, 8–13.

Goldstein, A. P. (1981). *Psychological skill training.* New York: Pergamon Press.

Heasley, B. (1974). *Auditory perceptual disorders and remediation.* Springfield, IL: Charles C Thomas.

Kramer, C. H., & Kramer, J. R. (1974). *Developing a therapeutic community.* Springfield, IL: Charles C Thomas.

Kuehrel, T. C., DeRisi, W. J., Lieberman, R. P., & Mosk, M. D. (1983). Treatment strategies that promoted deinstitutionalization of chronic mental patients. In W. P. Christian, G. T. Hannah, & T. J. Glahn (Eds.), *Deinstitutionalization: Strategies for effective transition of clients to the community.* New York: Plenum Press.

Levy, L. (1987). Psychosocial intervention and dementia, Part 1: State of the art, future directions. *Occupational Therapy in Mental Health,* 7(1) 68–107.

Lewis. S. C. (1979). *The mature years: A geriatric occupational therapy text.* Thorofare, NJ: Charles B. Slack.

Lieberman, R. P., Mueser, K. T., & Wallace, C. J. (1986). Social skills training for schizophrenic individuals at risk for relapse. *American Journal of Psychiatry, 143,* 523–526.

Magara, P. A., & DeSisto, M. (1981). A developmental treatment program for the chronic patient. *American Journal of Psychotherapy, 35,* 1.

Maslin, D. (1982). Rehabilitation training for community living skills: Concepts and techniques. *Occupational Therapy in Mental Health 2,* 33–49.

Mosey, A. (1973). *Activities therapy.* New York: Raven Press.

Paire, J. A., & Karney, R. J. (1984). The effectiveness of sensory stimulation for geropsychiatric inpatients. *American Journal of Occupational Therapy, 38*(8), 505–509.

Paul, G. & Lentz, R. (1977). *Psychosocial treatment of chronic mental patients: Milieu versus social learning programs.* Cambridge, MA: Harvard University Press.

Team Building in the Psychiatric Hospital

7

Suzanne Goren

The dual criteria for measuring the effectiveness of work teams are organizational performance (accomplishing the tasks for which they were created) and management of the team's own interpersonal process. Although these responsibilities are discrete, they are interrelated. When consensus on organizational mission and team goals is lacking, or when team members are unable to resolve ongoing conflicts, team performance inevitably suffers. Team building is an intervention into a team's process. It provides staff members with the opportunity to influence the quality of their work life by means of shared problem solving regarding goal setting, decision making, and conflict resolution. It is most often utilized at critical points in team development by newly created teams as a format for setting team goals and establishing process norms, or by established teams that have drifted to low task performance or are facing major organizational change.

Team building was employed as part of a larger attempt to transform the hospital from its historic role as a long-term, custodial institution to a discharge-oriented system geared to the rehabilitation of elderly patients. Effecting such transformation required significant change in widely held beliefs about patients' potential for self-governance and in the performance of all roles within the institution. If the rehabilitation model of treatment was to successfully replace custodial care, staff members' emphasis on "doing for" and "thinking for" patients, would have to be replaced by the attitudes and behaviors that support patients' taking responsibility for their own care and for making decisions. The decision to employ team building was a demonstration of the Institution's intention to develop a work environment that would support this goal. It was also symbolic of the commitment to solving organizational problems by participative problem solving, and recognition that staff members have untapped ability, the potential for growth, and the capacity for critical examination of the organizational culture.

Team building is a problem diagnosis and problem-solving workshop for team members, which provides them with a process for identifying their own issues and working productively toward their resolution. It is based on the assumptions that coordinated efforts of team members result in better outcomes than the effort of any one team member, and that team coordination can be improved through a shared workshop experience.

The participants in a team-building workshop consist of a work team charged with specific tasks, and a facilitator external to the system. The facilitator is responsible for gathering and organizing data about how the team operates, feeding such information back to team members, and helping the groups work together to prioritize the issues that have been raised, and to plan intervention and evaluation strategies. Despite pressure from team members for the "expert's" solution to problems, the facilitator concentrates on teaching a process of problem identification, agenda building, and decision making, which the team can use in the future, thereby empowering them to clarify and resolve their own problems.

Because team building was developed in the corporate world as a method of increasing the effectiveness of industrial teams, attempting this technique in a hospital is something of a cross-cultural transplant. Although much of the process is directly applicable to teams that plan and deliver health care services, certain elements that differentiate the two cultures must be considered. Corporations have profitability as a ready measure of organizational effectiveness. Nonprofit hospitals have no such clear cut criteria for assessing performance, and are burdened with regulatory restraints and diffusion of power emanating from many sources. In addition, they share the norms common to health care providers: the traditional medical model of service, differences in the values, focus, and languages of the health care professional and nonprofessional team members, and the impact of the institution's size, structure, and culture on the organization of its work.

Furthermore, when the hospital functions within a centrally administered bureaucracy of hospitals in which resistance to change is the norm, success in transforming one institution will disturb the equilibrium of the rest of the system. Unless the new social norms and operations are accepted as system-wide standards of practice, notable change in one hospital will make it a deviant among its institutional peers. One can expect that attempts will eventually be made to punish deviance by negative sanctions, and that the larger system will work toward returning the hospital to conformity with the status quo (Goren & Ottaway, 1985). Therefore, the administrator who originates change must be prepared to take those risks that will most likely accompany success, and to ensure as much as possible that change-maintaining mechanisms will be built into the overall strategy for change.

Team building with this institutions' staff was organized into five phases: contracting, data collection, feedback, agenda building/action planning, and follow-up.

CONTRACTING FOR TEAM BUILDING

The administrator who originates change bears the most personal risk of isolation and loss of support within the larger system. Falling to a less-favored position within the system results in less ability to provide the staff with the resources (money, staff positions, training, etc.) needed to maintain change. Therefore, the initial contracting for team building includes the facilitator's best estimate of the administrator's stomach for the risks associated with change, willingness to see the project through to its conclusion, and understanding that completion may lead to staff demands for action that had not been contemplated at the outset. Because no staff member can be expected to go further out on a limb than the top administrator is willing to go, authority for team building and permission for staff participation must come from the top administrator of the institution, and the contract is made with that person.

In this project, discussion of the contract included both what was sought as the outcome of the process, that is, open communication among team members and participation of all levels of staff in shared goal setting and decision making, and those factors that the facilitator saw as necessary to carry the process forward. These included the administrator's public commitment to the process, access to all of the staff identified as workshop participants, time enough to carry out the project, and an appropriate consulting fee.

In planning this team-building experience, it was agreed that each unit-based interdisciplinary team, including all staff assigned to the patient living unit on all shifts (generally around 20 persons) would be trained as a team. Team building was also carried out with the Clinical and Medical Care Committee, which included the Medical and Clinical Directors, the heads of all professional departments and clinical services, and the Executive Committee, which comprised the top management of the institution including the C.E.O. Subsequently, the newly formed Support Services Committee, which included the department heads of each maintainance, business, and food-service department, was also included. For the purposes of this discussion, all teams and committees are referred to as teams.

Participation of the highest level managerial staff, in this case the Executive Committee, is critical because this team is a visible model for others, and subordinates will look to them for support and approval of new team behaviors. For team building to be successful in a health care setting, it is essential to ensure the participation of those who are often excluded from decision making, those low in the hierarchy and close to patients, as well as those at the top, who often determine critical policies and procedures with limited knowledge of the work experience and work-related concerns of line staff. In the many-leveled hierarchy of the traditional hospital, staff usually have a general idea of the roles of others, but have little information about the pressures and constraints under which others work. Defining the unit team as broadly as possible provides the opportunity for everyone to participate in identifying the "crunches," those things that interfere with the ability to get the work done, and sets the stage for action planning to reduce or eliminate them (Hoffman, 1975).

DATA COLLECTION

The techniques of data collection vary, but the goal is always to identify the process issues that team members experience as obstacles to the accomplishment of the team's tasks. In this institution, information about the team's functioning was collected through individual and small-group interviews with staff, and by observation of the teams in action. Team members were asked for their perceptions of the task of their team, how well they work together, what they like most about their work, what they see as their biggest problem, what they do to handle it, and what kinds of changes they would like to see. The troublesome process issues were reported in detail in some of the interviews, at other times they became evident as they were played out throughout the team-building experience.

For example, concerning one team for which ongoing power struggles were the norm, the mental health aide who was described by co-workers as the leader of a powerful, dysfunctional subsystem, sent a message that she refused to participate. This was a clear challenge to the facilitator, as well as a replication of her ongoing challenge to her head nurse's authority. Her intention to boycott the team building created noticeable anxiety among team members. Some who had ceded much of their own power to her wondered aloud if they could proceed without her. With the facilitator's acknowledgement of the aide's importance to the team, and the assurance that team building could nevertheless proceed successfully without her, the team was able to move ahead.

The basic rule for data collection is the assurance of anonimity without confidentiality. The facilitator is interested only in information that the interviewee is willing to discuss during the team-building session. However, the authorship of all information is disguised. The facilitator is responsible for maintaining the focus of the interviews and for making sure that the ground rules for data collection are clear: the goal of the team building is improvement in the team's communication and ability to perform its assigned tasks; the purpose of the interview is obtaining information that will assist in moving toward that goal.

As might be expected, staff approached the interview sessions with varied degrees of circumspection. Some were relieved by the assurance that they would not be identified as the source of information that they divulged, others were reckless, apparently unaware of or insensitive to their potential vulnerability; still others were disappointed that the interviews were not going to provide an opportunity for unrestrained catharsis.

FEEDBACK

Prior to feeding the interview material back to each team, the facilitator synthesizes and summarizes data so that it offers a focused picture of the problems identified by the members, and an analysis of how team members are currently attempting to manage problems. Block's criteria for feedback are helpful here. These include restrict the focus—"to items that the group can control, that are clearly important to the organization, and that the organization has some commitment to working on."(Block, 1981, p. 168). The importance of these criteria is that they increase the likelihood of success by aligning the team's efforts for change with the direction in which the larger organization is heading, and they prevent futile efforts in areas beyond the scope of the teams' authority.

The ultimate purpose of feedback is team members' recognition of the scope of their authority, and their acceptance of responsibility for solving problems within their control.

The information gathered from interviews was organized according to the dominant themes that emerged when the data was sorted into categories. At the team's feedback meeting each interviewee received a memo identifying the themes. There were many positive appraisals of the quality of care provided and the relationships between direct care staff and their immediate supervisors. These were included in the memos as well as problems. Direct quotes were indicated by quotation marks without identifying sources.

During the feedback meeting, team members were asked to edit the memo by questioning and clarifying the interview data, and adding anything significant they thought had been omitted. Questions about the accuracy of the feedback were turned back to the team, and the material was retained only when one or more team members supported its inclusion. The result of such group editing was twofold: the introduction of open communication as a first step in problem identification and decision making, and the development of an agreed upon data base, which is accepted as a fair presentation of the current issues and concerns of the team.

During feedback sessions, there is a risk of undermining the first steps toward problem resolution. This most often occurs when the team and the facilitator agree on problem definitions that leave problem solving outside the team's control (for example, determining that raising team morale requires the institution's return to a custodial model of care), or when the group avoids discussion of difficult relationships that have a bearing on the problem. (Block, 1981). At times, feedback presents individuals with their first inkling that their own concerns are shared by others. Sometimes it covers information that team members already have, but which they have not dealt with directly. The feedback process facilitates taking ownership of problems, confronting issues, and openly communicating about them. In this institution, feedback sessions with several teams began with concerted efforts to promote the myth that staff had no power to change their work situation. However, discussion of the feedback data was a first step toward staff's perception of themselves as problem solvers and change agents.

In the feedback to the team mentioned earlier, the conflict among team members created an uproar among the allies of the absent aide, who insisted that we could not discuss this data without her. However, those who had described the issue during their interview, and had indicated their willingness to use team building to talk about it openly for the first time, took ownership of the data, insisting that the situation was accurately portrayed in the feedback memo and that they were committed to changing it. The feedback was a revelation to the head nurse, who learned to her surprise that most of her staff wanted her to take charge, and would support her efforts to do so. For members of the team, resisting mutiny and supporting legitimate authority, controlling the agenda, and dealing constructively with difficult material were empowering activities that made it possible to envision themselves as a more harmonious and constructive team.

The dominant themes throughout all the interviews were (a) concern about the changed goals of the hospital and resultant changes in expectations of the standards of care, (particularly as they related to the patients' self-determination and staff's control of patients' behavior) and (b) concern about the process of decision making and conflict resolution throughout the hospital.

GOALS

In general, institutional mission statements and goals are of minor interest to line staff because they are viewed as abstractions having no relationship to the daily work of the "little guys." In this setting, however, the staff was quite concerned about the hospital's direction, and about the changes that would accompany its transformation to an active treatment setting. At the time of team building, there was virtually unanimous agreement that the current quality of patient care was excellent, and there was a high level of commitment to maintaining this standard. Quite a few staff stated that they would feel comfortable entrusting members of their own families to the hospital, an assessment of the quality of care unusual in a public institution. Their deserved pride in the quality of their own work (assessed on the basis of norms for custodial care) served for some staff members as the rationale for resisting major change. A frequent statement among this staff was, "If it ain't broke, don't fix it!"

Nevertheless, despite fears that care would be compromised by moving patients into less desirable settings in the community, the consensus among many professional team members was that the institution was moving in the right direction. Some who had thought that discharge planning was unrealistic expressed relief that their earlier fears of "dumping" patients into the community had not been realized, and now saw the rehabilitation model more positively, "our patients deserve the opportunity to try it on the outside."

In general, resistance to a rehabilitative approach was most evident among staff nurses and mental health aides throughout the system, while the major advocates for change were rehabilitation and social-work staff. In those teams in which the conflict about goals was most evident, discipline-specific loyalties across team boundaries increased at the expense of team cohesiveness and performance. Another variation of team dysfunction was manifested by a team in which cohesiveness was based on staff's unanimous advocacy for continued custodial care. Here, the general agreement to oppose institutional changes led to sabotage of discharge plans and undermining of treatment programs. Some long-term employees defined defense of custodial care as patient advocacy, and described efforts to discharge patients as a violation of the hospital's historic promise to be the patients' permanent home. Among this group there were a few who were committed to loyalty to old ways of doing things simply because they had always been done that way; more commonly, the belief that the rehabilitation model could not succeed was based on low estimates of the patients' potential.

Organizational changes were a source of difficulty for the executive and clinical teams as well, because of members' ambivalence about the new approach to treatment. Some were clear about the differences between old and new ways of working, and were excited about the possibility of working in a less traditional and hierarchal system. Others stated that the change to a rehabilitative model was a change only on paper, and would alter only the number of rehabilitation staff, rather than treatment itself. A third contingent described themselves as not understanding the model, and as waiting for the Clinical Director to fully describe it so them.

Because the clinical staff at the management level generally had a working understanding of the differences between rehabilitation and custody, executives' requests for more information could be interpreted as covert resistance. Given the norms of a state bureaucracy, pseudoignorance can at times be a tactic for avoiding the risk of publicly identifying with a maverick C.E.O. Although clinical/executive team members agreed that they would be rewarded for their attempts to abandon the clinical approaches and management strategies associated with custodial care, there was concern that such a philosophy made the C.E.O.'s tenure uncertain, and that a replacement might very well be intolerant of the changes that were being initiated. As middle managers in an unpredictable system in which local top management turnover was high, executive committee members' strategies of keeping a low profile and offering covert resistance might indeed have been prudent methods of preserving their current status and protecting their future.

Fear of another sort also mitigated change in the hospital. With increased independence and improved ADL skills as the treatment focus, a shift from perceiving patients as stereotyped nursing home residents to active psychiatric patients would have to made. Such a shift was seen as especially dangerous by those staff members providing direct patient care. The staff expressed their insecurity regarding psychiatric patients, describing them as "more unpredictable, more stressful, and creating more crises" than geriatric patients. For them, change to active treatment implied that contradictory demands would be placed on them: on one hand, the expected loss of control of patients' behavior led them to see a need for increased use of repressive interventions including seclusion and restraint; at the same time, they would be expected to support patients' efforts at self-governance. Even those who described active work with psychogeriatric patients as "more interesting and more exciting" recognized these patients as "riskier" than a purely geriatric population, and some admitted to fear that the environment, which was without locked doors and enclosed nursing stations, would be inadequate to protect them from aggressive behavior.

DECISION MAKING

Decision making is frequently the arena in which hidden agendas and interpersonal conflicts are played out. The necessity of dealing with the same patient-related issues repetitively, inabiity of teams to make timely decisions, the length of meetings, and the lack of line nursing staff input into clinical decision making were identified as major obstacles to development and implementation of coherent treatment plans.

The wide range of opinion about how much might reasonably be expected of patients, ranging from: "Our system is repressive . . . patients are not encouraged to do enough for themselves," to: "You can't do much with them," ". . . Why bug old people? They've earned the right to sit" "When I'm old I want to be left alone," led to a lack of concensus about those decisions that had been made, and uneven efforts to implement treatment plans.

There was an estrangement among shifts, an ongoing struggle for power, control, and territorial rights. Despite efforts to provide continuity across shifts, staff on each tended to criticize the others for permissiveness (or rigidity), and did not experience themselves as part of a round-the-clock team. Several interviewees talked about one case, in which night staff in a case conference seminar carefully worked out a treatment plan for a diabetic patient who often rose in a belligerent, fugue state when awakened at the usual early morning hour. She was to be allowed to sleep until her natural waking hour, and her breakfast was to be kept warm by the day staff who were to ensure that she ate. Despite the participation of the C.E.O. and the Director of Nursing in the development of the plan, it was sabotaged by the day staff who allowed the meal to become cold (and hence inedible), rebuked the patient for sleeping late, and angrily stated that the plan represented "giving in to patients" who should conform to standard rules.

Delayed decision making and lack of commitment to decisions that have been made are commonly used tactics to avoid direct confrontation on sensitive issues. Frequently they are used as a screen to mask personal resistance to threatening changes in role expectations and in the balance of power among team members. As in most institutions, nurses' aides had the least formal education and the most limited behavioral repertoire for intervening with patients. Abandoning the familiar modes of custodial care would result in a significant loss of control for those team members whose status in the institution formerly depended on exercising unquestioned authority over patients, and enforcing inflexible institutional rules. Similarly, the physician's centrality and control would be reduced, and the influence of social work and rehabilitation increased if the present model were to be replaced by a discharge-oriented approach.

With unresolved patient care issues as ongoing issues, and concerns about potential changes in their own roles as a hidden agenda, teams consistently spent far more than the allotted team meeting time wrestling with treatment decisions. Staff complained that despite too many meetings which ran too long, they were always behind on scheduled case conferences. When the pressure of time or the need to coordinate their efforts with community agencies forced a decision, teams generally settled for the majority opinion. Subsequently, some of the minority contingent undermined the agreed upon plans by nonparticipation or by allying themselves with patients' resistance to change, while others called in administrators who could be counted on to be allies. The teams' inability to make decisions, and the feeling that one could never be sure of closure on any given issue was a source of generalized frustration.

Powerlessness and mystification were other themes that ran through all the data related to decision making. In speaking of team structure, Weisbord indicates that structure (i.e., division of labor) makes an enormous difference and is usually underrated. He suggests that the unhappiest teams are those where everybody has multiple skills and where there's no procedure for sorting out who should do what when (Weisbord, 1974). Unhappiness also exists in teams in which the lateral boundaries between skills are not at issue, but there is confusion in sorting out the level at which "who should do what when." At this institution, team members were unsure of which decisions they were actually authorized to make, and which should be referred upward, by which mechanism, to the administrative level.

Clinical managers were unsure of what caused the teams' paralysis, and stated that they stepped in to make decisions only because their subordinates could not act decisively. Clinical staff acknowledged that teams were generally perceived as "dysfunctional" by outsiders, and agreed that they were inefficient. Nevertheless, they were resentful that their decisions were frequently overridden, and that all really important decision making was reserved for the top administrative level at the hospital and for those above them in the central office. Nurses and mental health aides who provided daily care to patients felt disenfranchised, and complained of having little impact on decisions that affected their own work, that is, program changes, relocation of patients, staff assignments, and scheduling.

When asked for hypotheses about why "discussions go round and round and decisions are deferred" in their own team, executive team members suggested not wanting to bear the onus for making an unpopular decision, fear of making a mistake or of being seen as insensitive, and carrying on the State tradition of allowing a crisis to develop before taking action." They described an ongoing power struggle with the C.E.O., in which "she tries to make us responsible for making decisions . . . we try to push it back on her."

This kind of struggle exemplifies the play between the forces in the leader, forces in the subordinates, and forces in the system that exert significant influence on managerial style (Tanenbaum & Schmidt, 1958). Despite the C.E.O.'s expressed value system and her inclination toward sharing authority and responsibility, subordinates' personal management styles and prior socialization in the state mental health system (including top-down authoritarian management) made them reluctant to accept the challenge of shared authority and responsibility. Some simply did not believe her offer was authentic, believing that she controlled the group by making her preferred outcomes known. Others felt that control of the executive group would be ceded to the members as they decreased their need for authoritarian leadership and became more competent problem solvers.

AGENDA BUILDING/ACTION PLANNING

Teams used the feedback data to determine what the most pressing problems were, and the order in which they would deal with them. Because each team had identified decision making as problematic, the process of establishing priorities was used as a vehicle for teaching decision-making skills, that is, active listening, constructive feedback, brainstorming, and concensus building. Setting the first priority was the most difficult; after that the teams became more efficient as they worked past old habits of nonparticipation, disengagement, and pessimism.

Once the priorities had been set, each team worked on a plan of action to bring about desired change. Kurt Lewin's Force Field Analysis was used as the framework for action planning because it encourages development of strategies for maximizing systemic strengths and minimizing weaknesses, much as the rehabilitation approach does with individuals. For teams in which some members insisted that staff was impotent, others were able to identify the individuals and organizational structures that might assist in a change effort. Each team's action plan included a clear statement of the desired outcome, the steps that would be taken toward that outcome, staff member(s) accepting responsibility for each step, a target date for its completion, a monitor who would check the process of each step, and a mechanism for reporting progress back to the larger group.

As action planning proceeded, and team members learned a step-by-step series of problem-solving skills, most became more optimistic about the possibility of becoming change agents in their own system. However, there were some who could not be engaged in the process, who didn't believe change was possible or wanted to avoid it, or who were apathetic and simply let others do the work. The most imaginative among the active staff made the leap from being learners to envisioning a scenario in which they would work with patients to develop the skill and the courage for their own personal decision making.

FOLLOW-UP

Because team building was one of several change initiatives instituted at the hospital simultaneously, it is not possible to determine precisely what each contributed to the overall change effort. One outcome attributed to the team building was the reorganization of the Executive Committee into a new executive body, which combined the clinical and support services committees. Because this was a large group for decision making, each meeting began with the agenda-building process to ensure that all relevant issues were included. The length of meetings decreased as time limits were set and observed, and staff felt better about the meetings as they became more productive. Months later, members recommended reducing the numbers of staff involved. A level of trust had developed that allowed them to rely on representatives to present and negotiate their issues.

There was also a marked improvement in the level of trust among members of the Clinical–Medical Care Committee. Their committment to the process developed as communication opened up members who were able to take the risk of being candid with each other. Feedback to the facilitator several years after the project was completed, identified the change in this team as the catalyst for change in the support-services team, which became less fearful and distrustful and more productive.

Most teams reported change in the form of improved interdisciplinary relationships (particularly between the nursing and rehabilitation staffs), more efficient and participatory clinical decision making, and team members' increased sensitivity to the problems and constraints affecting others.

The team-specific outcomes were as varied as the teams themselves. Some reported attempts at change followed by backsliding into old practices, which they followed with further attempts to reestablish the new ways of working together. In one instance, team members felt that an influential member was passively thwarting the process. After confronting the issue and resolving it with the team member's participation, including his request for feedback about his nonproductive behavior, the team became much more effective.

One team reported no change at all as a result of the team building; at the other end of the continuum was the team that came to the follow-up meeting bearing a huge banner proudly proclaiming itself "Team IV—The Change Makers."

REFERENCES

Block, P. (1981). *Flawless consulting.* San Diego: University Associates.

Goren, S., & Ottaway, R. (1985). Why health care teams don't change: Chronicity and collusion. *Journal of Nursing Administration,* 15(7, 8), 9–17.

Hoffman, R. I. (1975). *Team building.* IBM: Unpublished internal document.

Weisbord, M. (1974). A mixed model for medical centers: Changing structure and behavior. In J. Adams (Ed.), *Theory and method in organization development: An evolutionary process.* Arlington, VA: National Institute for Applied Behavioral Science.

Tannenbaum, R., & Schmidt, W. (1958). How to choose a leadership pattern. *Harvard Business Review, 36,* 95–101.

8 Perspectives on Change

Assessment of the effects of change before a considerable amount of time has elapsed is a risky undertaking. It requires time for the glow of enthusiasm and conviction to settle, time to know which initiatives have sustained, which have not, and what in fact have been the long-term effects.

So, within the context of this understanding, we will examine the extent to which the established mission, goals, and objectives of this endeavor were met, describe some evidence of change in attitudes and expectations, and look at some other factors and outcomes.

THE MISSION: GOALS AND OBJECTIVES

As stated earlier, our overall mission was to provide a comprehensive treatment and rehabilitation program that would make it possible for patients to achieve their highest level of independent functioning in daily living activities, enable their adaptation to community living, and foster individual potential and self-determining behaviors. A concomitant purpose was to establish a total therapeutic community as the modus operandi of the institution, develop and maintain collaborative relationships with community agencies, offer, in concert with them, a spectrum of community-based service options and foster public understanding and support.

One philosophic tenet that influenced the priority sequencing of these goals and objectives was the belief that expectations set for patients must be congruent with the values and beliefs of the staff. The staff's attitude must be one that is ready to support and facilitate those behaviors and functions expected of patients. It was imperative therefore that changes in staff attitudes and values occur before significant change in patient care and treatment could be undertaken with any degree of anticipated success. A related value held that the structure and operations of an institution must foster those attitudes, behaviors, and social roles expected of staff and patients; that the institution's way of operating should enable the discovery and practice of new learning, of new ways of perceiving and functioning; that therefore the best forum for attitudinal change and staff education is in the daily administration and operations of the institution.

It was evident then that our first priority was to move toward the creation of a decentralized, horizontal, participatory management system; the generation of an open system of communication and development of a total therapeutic community. In terms of staff functioning and management procedures, the goals of open communication and participatory management were successfully achieved. Progress of patients in these areas was less marked. Although there was evidence of a diminishing sense of helplessness among patients, on the average, they were not understandably ready to fully engage in open communication or participatory decision making. There were of course some notable exceptions, especially among the transitional living group and the core group of the Patient Council. Although work with this latter group had created a structure and procedure for a more empowered Council, recruitment of others to join them was a slow and cautious process.

For some of these same reasons, the development of a total therapeutic community moved slowly. Full implementation of this endeavor requires the active engagement of patients and the habitual passive patterns from years of illness and institutionalization are relinquished slowly and cautiously. It is reasonable to expect that the level of participation for many of these patients will increase with time and with continued support for trying out new behaviors. It is encouraging to know that those mentally ill elderly now being admitted directly from the community will have the benefit of an environment that supports and sustains functional, productive values and behaviors and expects early return to the community.

Closely related to the above as a force in shaping attitudes and behaviors is the nature of the nonhuman environment. The goal of establishing a responsive, clarifying physical environment was, as stated earlier, based on the belief that the nature and characteristics of the physical environment impacts in a positive or negative way, the responses of patients and staff to performance expectations. Chapter 4 describes in part how this goal was conceptualized and achieved.

All patient living areas, staff offices, and most congregate areas were refurbished and redecorated. Patient living and working areas were redesigned to compensate as much as possible for the patients' perceptual and functional losses. Patient rooms were redone to eliminate the institutional look and achieve an individualized, comfortable, home-like atmosphere. Each floor was distinguished by its unique style of furnishings and decor, such as early American, Provincial, and the like. Attractive, graphic designs were painted on long corridor walls and large wall spaces to diminish the sense of vastness as well as to provide directional cues. The routines, schedules, and other daily operations of each patient living unit were planned and carried out according to the rehabilitation purpose of each floor and thus to elicit and support the expected behaviors and functioning of patients and staff. This goal was certainly achieved and with only moderate cost to the system.

A vigorous and comprehensive in-service education program for all staff was critical to the success of our mission. It is important to emphasize here that both the processes of changing communication and management patterns and the changed, new environment provided rich learning experiences for staff and patients and created a culture that nourished the learning and practice of new behaviors. Such in vivo experience, we believe, is the finest of education modules.

The team building program described in Chapter 7 extended over a period of approximately 18 months and was a top priority. This experiential learning focused on teaching staff a process for identifying and resolving problems while simultaneously providing a safe "laboratory" for trying out new behaviors, confronting issues, putting things on the table, learning about interdependence, self-advocacy, the significant other, and empowerment. In other words, learning what an authentic team and team membership was all about. Such learning translated into noticeably improved team functioning and significant change in staff attitudes and involvement.

It is well known that the success of most any endeavor depends on commitment of those who will be expected to carry out the mission. Staff's acceptance of the changes being initiated was conseqently critical to the outcome of our mission. Staff development and education programs were thus aimed at enabling all staff at all levels to understand the overall mission and its rationale as well as each phase of the plan and to teach them the skills they would need as participants and implementors. It has been said that it is not so much the change that generates fear, anxiety, and thus resistance as it is the uncertainty that surrounds any change. Not being able to predict, discovering that one's learned cause and effect equations are not necessarily applicable, and simply not knowing, are disturbing feeling states. Planning and structuring the change process provides some sense of being in some control. Staff education and training initiatives that both enable understanding and provide the related skill learning give an added sense of control, a sense of probable competence in managing the process.

Such learning was provided for all aspects of this project and typically presented and adjusted so that it was relevant and had meaning for all staff at all levels. The impact of the staff development program on staff morale will be addressed later. Some additional measures of the success of this endeavor is evident in the fact that it was possible to move and relocate more than 50 patients, move many staff with related changes in their roles and responsibilities without a single altercation or even moderately serious problem.

Designing and implementing the plan for patient treatment and rehabilitation was begun only after changes in management and communication processes of the institution were in place and operating. The patient-services initiative involved developing an interdisciplinary functional skills-assessment training for each treatment team in the collaborative assessment procedure, obtaining a team assessment on every patient, aggregating and analyzing data, creating six functionally homogeneous patient living units based on data, relocating patients and staff accordingly, training teams to plan and implement treatment and rehabilitation programs congruent with the level of functioning and expected outcomes of their unit, planning and opening a 32-bed short-term, acute admissions unit.

Three functional levels were established. One transitional living unit of 22 beds was designed to prepare patients for entry into the community, two intermediate level units were established for 56 patients for whom the goal was progress into the transitional living unit or discharge to supervised care in the community. Four basic level units for 91 patients were developed. These units contained the lowest functioning patients and had as their goal, the progression of the patient to an intermediate level of functioning or enabling the patient to develop those behaviors and functions that would qualify them as acceptable candidates for admission to a proprietary skilled nursing or intermediate care facility. Contract agreements were developed with nursing homes that include our agreement to provide a staff training program, consultation and short-term admissions in exchange for placements for our patients.

Nine months after these programs were in place, six patients had been discharged from the transitional unit to boarding homes, a group home, and a senior citizens residence. The number of basic units had been reduced to two, and three intermediate level units had been created.

By the end of the year, 10 patients had been discharged to boarding or group homes, three returned to their families, and 102 patients were discharged to proprietary nursing homes. Admissions had risen accordingly and the level of functioning significantly improved. The short-term acute unit was providing a comprehensive evaluation and diagnosis service, an outreach service, and triage. It seems reasonable to attribute the smooth transition of these endeavors to the management changes and staff education that preceded them.

Full accreditation as a psychiatric hospital was received from the Joint Commission on Accreditation of Health Organization (JCAHO) and the federal government and we began the final phase of our project. A coalition was established with state and local community agencies to plan for the continuity of care of the elderly. Contract agreements with agencies were finalized and plans for a community-based day treatment center and a housing program were completed. These programs aimed at providing a critical transition from hospitalization to community living, reducing recidivism, deterring or postponing the need for hospitalization and providing appropriate housing for those for whom family living was not an option. Unfortunately a change in state administration and priorities redirected funding and these initiatives were not implemented.

CHANGING ATTITUDES AND EXPECTATIONS

Perhaps one of the most apparent indicators of staff satisfaction and high morale was the impressive reduction in staff turnover. However, a number of other outcomes can be identified as evidence of changed attitudes and expectations.

One of the most pervasive set of attitudes, especially among nursing staff related to the belief that quality nursing care was characterized by doing for the patient, that old people had earned the right to be taken care of, and that patients should not be expected to be active or independent. During the early phase of our work, staff was exceedingly protective of the patient, defending their right to be cared for and "not pressed to be active." Such alliances between patients and staff were too frequent and obviously presented some complex and difficult clinical issues. Over time however, there began to be more and more references to and discussions about improved patient functioning and independence. Only seldom did one hear statements about the rights of patients to be sedentary and dependent and there was a discernible diminution in the frequency of staff's overt or covert support of such behaviors. For example, the content of morning rounds no longer centered around incidents of patients decompensating because of pressures to perform or from the "stress of expectations." Rather, staff more and more reported on the achievement of patients, looked for and received approbation from peers for having enabled a patient to achieve.

There was a surge of interest in the development of patient programs and activities. New and innovative ideas began to be suggested with competition between units and a beginning sense of ownership of programs and missions.

There were changes in perspectives and behaviors regarding disciplinary roles and responsibilities. Initial fears and defensiveness gave way at first to tolerance, then to increasing clarification of unique expertise and respect for one another. Interdisciplinary staff education, especially the team building was successful in breaking down old barriers between disciplines and giving meaning to the collaborative dynamic of a team and the uniqueness of each member.

The increasing attendance at the open community meetings, fewer and fewer requests for management to intervene, and the recommendation of the large and initially suspicious executive committee that its numbers should be reduced, reflected a growing change in staff attitudes and expectations.

Accreditation surveyors and visitors alike commented again and again about the staff's obvious pride in the institution and what it was contributing to the welfare of patients. What was observable was staff's eagerness to show visitors around, their positive comments, sense of purposeful work, and lack of complaint while acknowledging that much still needed to be accomplished. A frequent comment of management and line staff was "I would have no reservations about being a patient here."

The "mainstreaming" of night staff paid dividends in many ways. The staff education seminars and conferences, the involvement of top administrators and department heads during night hours added to staff's understanding of patients, enlisted them in the daily operations of the facility and in the clinical management of patients. Although there continued to be differences of opinion and territorial struggles, these became less frequent and more out in the open where they could be addressed. The quality of patient care and treatment during the night hours was significantly enhanced as was the substance of the communication and interaction between shifts.

Because of limited experience with psychiatric patients, many staff were fearful and questioned their ability to manage those patients who would be admitted as a result of the change in mission. There was strong pressure for the creation of seclusion rooms and for a policy of locked doors. In addition to a staff education module that dealt with understanding and managing the geropsychiatric patient, the arrival on staff of clinical nurse specialists went a long way toward allaying anxiety. The expertise and role modeling provided by these professionals made a significant difference. Locked doors and seclusion rooms disappeared from agendas.

As the interdisciplinary functional skill-assessment methodology was implemented, inappropriate referrals from treatment teams became less and less frequent and ultimately disappeared as a problem. There was also a marked reduction in the stalemates that frequently occurred regarding the transfer of a patient from one floor to another. Such incidents had become so frequent and so intransigent that an independent committee had been established to make transfer decisions. Subsequent to staff training and implementation of the Functional Skill Assessment-Procedures, the committee was no longer needed and it was disbanded.

Changes in patient attitudes and expectations moved more slowly, in part because changes in their programs and daily living routines were implemented later, and in part because they had been well socialized into the traditional role of patient. Nevertheless, evidence of altering expectations could be seen in their more active involvement in programs, the growing popularity of their volunteer service club, proactive agendas for the council and the red-letter day when they challenged top management regarding a decision that altered space in the chapel about which they had not been consulted. Reduction in the number of beds in the basic units was the result not only of the discharge of patients to nursing homes but also because of the increasing progress of patients toward a higher level of overall functioning.

OTHER CONCLUSIONS

At the start of our project we hypothesized that in the last analysis, it would prove to be a cost-effective endeavor. It seems prudent therefore to examine this expectation. Although the physical environment had been completely refurbished and redecorated and the number and expertise of professional staff more than doubled, our annual per capita costs were impressively lower than other state institutions, even among those with a lower bed capacity. In 1987, for example, our annual per capita costs were approximately 35% below the average institutional costs to the system as a whole. Our daily per capita of $107.33 was noteworthy when compared with the range of $191.46 to $132.75 for other institutions with a high of $191.46 to a low of $132.75.

Accreditation as a psychiatric hospital rather than a nursing home significantly increased the rate of reimbursement. More than one half of the total cost of operation was met by such revenue. Most significant perhaps, was that mental health dollars that had previously gone to provide nursing home care were now freed and available for the care and treatment of the mentally ill.

It is remarkable that during this period of significant change in staff roles and responsibilities, labor and management enjoyed a special relationship, one characterized by mutual respect, open communication, and collaboration.

One truth has emerged from this experience: those elements that nurture competence are the same for staff as they are for patients. The total environment, its human and nonhuman characteristics and dynamics, without question, determine outcome. Another understanding that emerged was how very important it is to ensure that there is a system of support for taking a chance, risking a new discovery. Top authority must make clear its willingness and ability to absorb a glitch, a goof, or an error. It must be obvious that one is not alone, out on a limb, but rather that the process of exploring new territory is a shared collaborative experience.

Growth and change have their own time. What we have demonstrated in this limited time is that achievement of high-quality patient care and treatment in a state psychiatric system is indeed possible. Sustaining that quality in a bureaucracy over a significant period of time is another matter and only time will answer our question. What is knowable now is perhaps best expressed by a staff member who commented, "We now know what quality is all about. We now know that it can be done and no matter what may happen, we will carry that knowing with us for the rest of our lives."

INDEX